THE NEW ATKINS MADE EASY

COLETTE HEIMOWITZ

ALSO AVAILABLE:

New Atkins for a New You

The New Atkins New You Cookbook

THE *NEW* ATKINS

MADE EASY

A FASTER, SIMPLER WAY to SHED WEIGHT and FEEL GREAT—STARTING TODAY!

COLETTE HEIMOWITZ

Vermilion
LONDON

10 9 8

First published in the United Kingdom in 2014 by Vermilion, an imprint of Ebury Publishing
A Random House Group company
First published in the United States by Touchstone, a division of Simon & Schuster, Inc. in 2013

The Random House Group Limited Reg. No. 954009

Addresses for companies within the Random House Group can be found at www.randomhouse.co.uk

Penguin Random House is committed to a sustainable future for our business, our readers and our planet. This book is made from Forest Stewardship Council® certified paper.

MIX
Paper from
responsible sources
FSC® C018179

Printed and bound in Great Britain by Clays Ltd, St Ives plc

ISBN 9780091954918

To buy books by your favourite authors and register for offers visit www.randomhouse.co.uk

The information in this book has been compiled by way of general guidance in relation to the specific subjects addressed, but is not a substitute and not to be relied on for medical, healthcare, pharmaceutical or other professional advice on specific circumstances and in specific locations. So far as the author is aware the information given is correct and up to date as at January 2014. Practice, laws and regulations all change, and the reader should obtain up to date professional advice on any such issues. The author and publishers disclaim, as far as the law allows, any liability arising directly or indirectly from the use, or misuse, of the information contained in this book.

Contents

PART III: IT'S ALL ABOUT FOOD

PART IV: RECIPES

Index of Week-at-a-Glance Meal Plans

Introduction

Many books have been written about the Atkins Diet. And no wonder! The world's most famous diet is famously effective. Year after year, millions of people achieve dramatic results. In more than 110 papers published in peer-reviewed journals, eating the Atkins way has been scientifically proven to produce both sustained weight loss and robust health improvements. No other weight-loss programme comes close to this number. Last, but far from least, the Atkins Diet is delicious and nutritious.

We're proud of this record of accomplishment, but as part of our ongoing objective to help people lose weight and keep it off, we're always working to enhance the Atkins experience. That's why we regularly ask Atkins followers for input on how to improve the programme. As part of that research, we also speak to would-be dieters about why they haven't tried Atkins yet and what would make them consider doing so.

What have we learned? Some people tell us that the programme seems complicated, that they're too busy to cook, or that low-carb cooking seems to require lots of different ingredients. Some aren't sure what Net Carbs are or how to count them. Others don't understand the need for four phases and/or how to move from one to the next. Finally, there's the misconception that Atkins is about eating no carbs, which would be hard to sustain and hardly healthy. Ouch! In part, this confusion exists because the experience of doing Atkins is fundamentally different from that of other weight-loss diets.

Nonetheless, we also clearly need to do a better job of communicating what Atkins is, why it works, and which foods you do and don't eat. People want a stripped-down approach that tells them how to use Atkins simply and easily without having to expend a lot of energy thinking about it. The hectic pace of contemporary life, compounded by the need to juggle work and family responsibilities, means most people have less time than ever to plan meals, shop, cook, and track their food intake.

Therein lies the purpose (and the heart) of *The New Atkins Made Easy*: to make the programme easier than ever before, both to understand and to follow. And that begins with how to get started – today. Getting meals on the table faster and easier is central to this objective. You should be able to pick up this book, head right out to the supermarket for a few supplies, and start your transformation the same day. No hassle, no fuss – just rapid results. The Atkins range of low-carb foods, including bars, shakes, crackers, and low-carb pasta, also makes it easier than ever to do Atkins.

EASY TO UNDERSTAND

The basic principles upon which Atkins is based are surprisingly simple; as are the steps you follow to achieve results. In a nutshell, here's how Atkins works:

- You eat a bit more protein – think chicken, fish, seafood, pork, beef, and tofu; more olive oil, butter, avocado, and other delectable fats that give food flavour; and lots of leafy greens and other vegetables.
- You initially hold off on higher-carb vegetables, as well as fruit and wholegrains.
- You omit starchy, sugary carbohydrate foods low in nutrients, such as bagels and sweetened breakfast cereals.

With these few simple changes your body burns its own fat for energy, while suppressing your appetite and eliminating cravings. The result? You lose the fat on your tummy, bum, hips, and elsewhere, all without undue hunger.

The power of Atkins is based on this remarkable but simple process that shifts your body from burning primarily carbohydrates for energy to burning primarily fat. In Chapter 1, we'll explore how you can quickly and easily make your metabolism work with you rather than resist you at every turn.

EASY TO DO

With this book in hand along with a supply of delicious Atkins bars, shakes, crackers, and low-carb pasta, you'll have all the tools you'll need to get going on your weight-loss journey, including:

- Step-by-step visuals that show which foods to add back into your diet and when, to help simplify the path to success
- Simplified meal plans for breakfast, lunch, dinner, and snacks, using everyday store cupboard items, and complete with shopping lists
- Easy and tasty low-carb recipes that use a minimum of ingredients.

You'll also learn how to:

- Scour the supermarket for Atkins-friendly options – more appear every day
- Modify family meals to make them Atkins friendly
- Put together a delicious low-carb menu without breaking the bank
- Manoeuvre through the maze of eating out by identifying which foods you can eat in different kinds of restaurants, as well as in fast-food places, and even at food stalls
- Prepare a strategy – ahead of time – to help stop a binge in its tracks
- Get the most out of your digital or printed food journal
- Use online resources and mobile apps such as the Atkins Carb Counter and Acceptable Foods Lists and meal plans for each phase.

ATKINS YOUR WAY

Another way in which we've made Atkins easier is by enabling you to customise it to your needs and the responses of your body. For example, you may prefer to lose most of your weight in the first phase of the programme. Or you may choose instead to move quickly through the first phase, begin to introduce greater food variety, and lose most of your weight in the second phase. The trade-off may be slightly slower weight loss. Decide which works better for you, and then follow the road map for that path. Whether you opt for the Fast Track or the Slow and Steady approach, you'll find all the details you need to succeed in the following chapters.

With these added features, you'll find it easy to achieve your weight-loss goal. How can I be so sure? Because I've seen it work for thousands of people just like you. I know that every weight-loss programme makes such promises. But in this case the evidence is undeniable. You could lose up to 7 kg (15 lb) in the first two weeks. (Obviously, results vary based on your body type, lifestyle, and other factors.) Yes, that's right, about a pound a day! It's a simple, delectable way of eating that you can follow not just for a few weeks, but for the rest of your life.

HOW ATKINS IS DIFFERENT

I'm not the only one singing the praises of the Atkins Diet. Millions of people around the world have opted for this programme and have an impressive track record of success. Here's how Atkins is different from other leading diets:

- *You'll see results quickly*. After just a few days, your clothes will begin to fit better. Talk about motivation!
- *You're never hungry*. Even as you cut down on carbohydrates (or carbs, as we usually refer to them), you eat every few hours. Three meals and two snacks a day mean no torturous between-meal tummy rumbling and no uncontrollable appetite at the next meal.
- *The food is delicious*. The quality and variety of food on Atkins is truly unparalleled. There's no way you'll stay with any dietary plan, no matter what the promised benefits, for more than a few weeks

if the food is tasteless and you're restricted to minuscule portions. Where else can you have a cheese omelette with a side of salsa for breakfast, a chef's salad topped with grilled chicken and blue cheese dressing for lunch, and grilled salmon with creamed spinach and sliced tomatoes for dinner? And then there are two yummy snacks, perhaps half an avocado in the morning and a chocolate shake mid-afternoon. Believe it or not, even with all this food you'll still lose weight!

- *You don't have to exercise to lose weight.* Though it's a good idea for other reasons, you don't have to engage in physical activity to get the benefits of the Atkins Diet.
- *Fat is not forbidden.* Eliminate empty carbs, and there's no problem eating healthy fats such as olive oil, avocados, high-oleic safflower oil, and flaxseed oil. Amazing but true: the fat you eat actually helps you burn the fat on your body.
- *It's affordable.* Poultry, eggs, burgers, and other inexpensive items are perfectly acceptable sources of protein. If you wish, confine your protein choices to fish or even vegetable sources of protein. The Atkins programme is incredibly flexible.
- *You'll still eat plenty of veggies.* While you'll ditch starchy and sugary processed foods, Atkins is not and never has been about no carbs. Atkins recommends a minimum of six servings of vegetables a day (and, depending on which vegetables you choose, you might actually get up to 12 servings). This exceeds the current NHS five-a-day dietary guidelines. Those vegetables will also give you lots of health-promoting fibre, antioxidants, and more.
- *It's easy to stick to Atkins.* The process of gradually reintroducing carbohydrate foods while continuing to shed pounds (and, later, maintaining weight loss) is the key to lasting success with Atkins. It's why so many people consider themselves "Atkins loyalists" who have made the programme part of their lifestyle.
- *Atkins is good for your health.* Study after study shows that eating a low-carb diet improves your cholesterol profile and blood-sugar levels, as well as other health markers. Following a low-carb lifestyle can also reverse metabolic syndrome and even Type 2 diabetes.

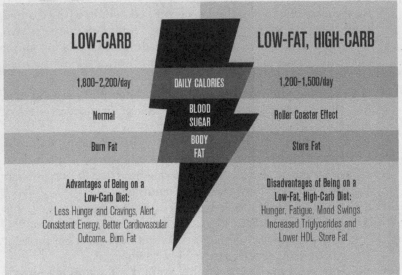

ADVANTAGES OF EATING LOW CARB

LOW-CARB		LOW-FAT, HIGH-CARB
1,800–2,200/day	DAILY CALORIES	1,200–1,500/day
Normal	BLOOD SUGAR	Roller Coaster Effect
Burn Fat	BODY FAT	Store Fat

Advantages of Being on a Low-Carb Diet:
Less Hunger and Cravings, Alert, Consistent Energy, Better Cardiovascular Outcome, Burn Fat

Disadvantages of Being on a Low-Fat, High-Carb Diet:
Hunger, Fatigue, Mood Swings, Increased Triglycerides and Lower HDL, Store Fat

ABOUT ME

I spent the first 10 years of my nutrition career counselling thousands of patients in doctors' offices in the New York City area on diet and lifestyle changes. In my next 20 years as a nutritionist I've been employed in one capacity or another by Atkins. For five years at the Atkins Centre I worked one-on-one with thousands of patients to help them slim down and deal with health problems. And for the following 15 years at Atkins Nutritionals, I've observed and advised many thousands of members of the Atkins community online in their weight-control efforts. I think it's fair to say that when it comes to eating habits and weight reduction, I've seen and heard it all. Now I'm excited at the opportunity to be your coach as you transform yourself into the new you. And, as always, you can communicate with me through my blog on atkins.com.

LET'S GET STARTED

If you're new to Atkins, welcome aboard. And if this is not the first time you've embarked on the programme, I promise that you'll find it easier than before. In either case, I'll repeat my original promise: try Atkins and you will lose weight.

All you have to lose are those pesky extra pounds. But what you have to gain is huge: for starters, a slimmer figure, renewed energy, confidence, a sense of being in control, and self-respect – and maybe even a whole new wardrobe. Plus stay with Atkins once you banish your extra pounds and you'll enjoy permanent weight control and enhanced health. Your new way of eating will let the new you emerge! Remember, I'll be with you every step of the way. Now turn the page and let's get down to business.

PART I

WHAT YOU NEED TO KNOW

CHAPTER 1

HOW ATKINS WORKS

Now that you know how easy, effective, and delicious Atkins is, I'm sure you're eager to get going ASAP, but hold on for just a moment. To get fabulous results and get them fast, you need to understand a few basics about how your body turns food into energy – the process called metabolism – and how that impacts on weight loss. Some of that energy is used immediately and the rest is stored. Whether you're brushing your teeth or running to catch a bus, your body draws on that stored energy. In addition to these conscious actions, countless other functions, including breathing, pumping blood through your body, digestion, and powering your brain cells, also call on your energy stores.

Carbohydrates and fats are the body's two sources of fuel. A low-fat diet is inevitably high in carbs, and when you take in more carbs than your body needs, it stores excess carbs as fat. Yes, sugar and other carbs convert to fat! That's one reason it's so hard to lose weight and keep it off on a low-fat diet. You have to cut back drastically on calories or you'll never burn your body fat. As a result, you're famished much of the time, and not many people can tolerate that for long. If you've tried low-fat weight-loss diets in the past, you know exactly what I'm talking about. However, if you restrict carbs sufficiently, as you do on Atkins, your body switches to its backup fuel, fat. Doing Atkins rebalances the ratio of fat to carbohydrate, transforming your metabolism from one that stores fat to one that burns fat. And when you're burning both dietary and body fat, you lose weight. That's the Atkins paradox: you can eat more fat, but that doesn't make you fat. In fact, as long as you control your carb intake, eating delicious fatty foods such as avocado and olive oil enables you to slim down. And once you reach a good weight for your height, body type, and age, this metabolic shift will continue to keep you slim. But the good news doesn't end there: burning fat can also usually stop metabolic syndrome, otherwise known as pre-diabetes, in its tracks, and can even reverse Type 2 diabetes.

IGNITE YOUR FAT-BURNING ENGINE

To understand how shifting to a fat metabolism results in weight loss, it helps to compare your body to a hybrid car. When the electricity stored in the engine battery is used up, the car automatically switches over to burning petrol. Likewise, your body always burns carbs before fat for energy. But when the carbs (in the form of blood sugar) are used up, your body switches over to burning fat for energy. This dual-fuel metabolism enabled our ancient ancestors to survive when food was scarce. But today, because most of us eat too much – or at least too many carbs – there's rarely or never a need to use our backup fuel.

So how do you help your body make the switch? Significantly cut back on your carb intake, and bingo – your fat metabolism kicks in. This is the essence of the Atkins Diet: control carbs to burn fat. If this sounds like hocus-pocus, remember that a large and ever-growing body of scientific research supports not just the efficacy of the low-carb approach, but also its safety. For more on the fat-burning metabolism and the research that supports it, see the Afterword, written by Jeff S. Volek, PhD, RD, on page 263.

GET OFF THE BLOOD SUGAR ROLLER COASTER

Have you ever eaten a high-carb meal – think about Christmas lunch – only to find yourself craving another serving of pudding topped with vanilla ice cream a few hours later? Or maybe you eat a breakfast consisting of cold cereal (often containing a lot of added sugar) and milk (full of natural sugar), a glass of orange juice (liquid sugar), and a cup of tea or coffee with a few more teaspoons of sugar. This

THE EFFECTS OF EATING A HIGH-CARB DIET

High-Carb Intake Results in Fat Storage:

INCREASES FAT STORAGE

STOP FAT BURNING

blood sugar spikes, which leads to...

Eating a lot of carbs leads to...

insulin spikes, which stop fat burning, which...

SPIKE IN BLOOD SUGAR

HIGH CARB INTAKE

THE EFFECTS OF EATING A LOW-CARB DIET

Low-Carb Intake Increases Fat Burning:

LOW-CARB INTAKE

NORMAL BLOOD SUGAR

Eating a low-carb diet leads to...

normal insulin levels, so your body can burn fat, which...

normal blood sugar levels, which leads to...

SHRINKS FAT CELLS

INCREASES FAT BURNING

CARB ROLLER COASTER

 ## CARB BALANCE

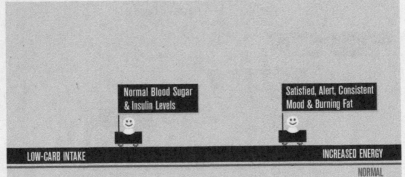

high-carb combination quickly boosts your blood-sugar level, stimulating the release of insulin to transport the sugar to your body's cells. This perfectly normal process keeps your blood-sugar level within a safe range.

If you're young, fit, and have no predisposition to blood-sugar issues, you may be able to get away with eating this way for years. (Or not – sad to say, since more and more children are developing high blood sugar and even Type 2 diabetes.) If insulin overcompensates, after a couple of hours your blood-sugar level drops quickly and precipitously. You feel sleepy, jittery, or unable to concentrate. Your body's response to this energy drain is to crave another high-sugar, high-starch, energy-boosting meal or snack. Welcome to the blood sugar roller coaster.

So you give in and have another sweetened cup of coffee or tea to rev up your engine, perhaps accompanied by a biscuit or a muffin. And the process starts all over again! You can see why I compare these rapid shifts between energy highs and lows to a roller-coaster ride. But getting off the roller coaster is easy – and I suspect you already know how. By controlling your carb intake and eating high-fibre carb foods with proteins and fats, you smooth out the wild swings and keep your blood sugar on an even keel. By minimising periods of low blood sugar, which triggers hunger for all the wrong foods, you'll find it easy to stay in control and not overeat. And, thanks to this new-found sense of control, you begin to shed pounds. That's why Atkins is so effective.

SUGAR AND YOUR HEALTH

Eating processed foods full of sugar harms you in two ways. First, obviously, you're adding empty carbs to your diet. And you're probably also not eating enough foods full of the vitamins, minerals, antioxidants, and fibre that help keep you healthy. We've long known that sugar intake promotes tooth decay and obesity, but study after study also directly links the intake of excess sugar to an increased risk of cancer, diabetes, gastrointestinal problems, eye diseases, osteoporosis, coronary heart disease, and other inflammatory diseases. Excess sugar also appears to affect the brain and has been implicated in poor memory formation, learning disabilities, depression, and even dementia. As you zero in on your goal weight, reducing your risk of all these conditions is also a powerful motivator for continuing to avoid added sugar whenever possible. Boxes throughout this book detail the dangers of added sugar in all its forms and point out where it lurks and what to substitute for it.

THE SKINNY ON CARBS

You know fat when you see it. Butter? Check. Olive oil? Check. Ditto with protein, although animal protein such as chicken, salmon, and the like, may spring to mind before lentils, tofu, and other vegetable sources. But I suspect some of you may be scratching your head and saying, "So what are carbs anyway?" Here's what you need to know:

- Carbs are found in all plant foods, including grains, cereals, potatoes, bread, and pasta. And everyone knows that sugar, which comes from plants, is packed with carbs. But all vegetables, from rocket to courgettes, and all fruits are also carb foods.
- Carb counts of different foods vary enormously. Berries are relatively low in carbs, for example, while bananas are at the other end of the spectrum. Likewise, salad leaves barely register on the carb scale, but potatoes and other starchy veg, such as peas, are much higher in carbs.
- Lettuce, spinach, and other leafy greens, along with dozens of other low-carb vegetables – we call them "foundation vegetables" to distinguish them from starchy vegetables – make up most of your initial carb intake on the Atkins Diet. (See pages 32–4 for more details.)
- The amount of carbs (as well as of protein and fat) in any food is measured in grams.
- Usually the higher the number of grams of carbs per serving, the faster and greater the impact on your blood sugar.
- Removing the fibre from food, as is the case with most fruit juices, white flour and other refined grain products, effectively raises the impact on blood sugar. It's preferable to eat whole fruit and brown rice and other wholegrains.
- Dairy products also contain some carbs, in the form of milk sugars.

- Carbs show up in some shellfish as well, although not in finned fish. (See page 30 for more on shellfish.)

THE CORE CARBS

It's important to understand that Atkins is not about eliminating all carbs. But there are some carb foods you'll avoid and others you'll eliminate initially. Early in the programme, you'll focus on certain foods that will continue to be the core of the New Atkins Diet as you increase and broaden your carb intake over time. The quality of the carbs you eat is as important as the quantity. Initially, you'll significantly lower your carb intake and you'll eat primarily wholegrain carbohydrates, including as many non-starchy vegetables as possible. You can also have most Atkins bars, shakes, crackers and, eventually, low-carb pasta. As you get closer to your goal weight, you'll reintroduce other high-fibre carbs, in a certain order, following the Carb Ladder (page 14).

THE SCOOP ON SUGAR: FAT TOOK THE HIT FOR SUGAR

For decades, fat was considered the main culprit in the obesity epidemic. We ate low-fat biscuits and drank skimmed milk, but our waistlines continued to expand. The real culprit, sugar, was hiding in plain sight in many so-called healthy foods and beverages.

But today nutritionists and doctors have named sugar as a major cause of the obesity epidemic – something we at Atkins have been saying for decades. The typical Brit now eats a staggering 30 kg (66 lb) of added sugars (including table sugar, high fructose corn syrup, and other caloric sweeteners) a year. And that's on top of the naturally occurring sugar we consume in fruits, vegetables, grains, dairy products, and other foods.

THE IMPORTANCE OF PROTEIN

Protein contains the amino acids that are the building blocks from which your body preserves existing (and forms new) muscle tissue, flesh, and nerves. Among the other functions enabled by this protein powerhouse are:

- Keeping warm
- Blood clotting
- Healthy brain function
- Manufacturing hormones, enzymes, and antibodies
- Maintaining an alkali/acid balance.

Eating an optimal amount of protein (and fat) while cutting down on carbs accomplishes a number of things, including:

- Satiating you, so you feel pleasantly full
- Moderating your blood-sugar level, helping tame your appetite for several hours
- Protecting muscle, so you shed only fat pounds once you've eliminated excess fluid in the first few days of the programme.

In no way is Atkins a high-protein diet. Guidelines call for 115–175 g (4–6 oz) cooked weight of protein foods at each meal. A petite, desk-bound woman might be satisfied with 115 g (4 oz), while an active guy might aim for 175 g (6 oz). (A very big guy might even want 225 g (8 oz).) But you won't have to weigh protein servings. Just compare them to certain common objects and pretty soon you'll be able to judge protein and other food portions accurately. (See "Portion Control" on page 49.) Your daily intake of protein foods will range 340–500 g (12–18 oz) cooked weight a day.

DIETARY FAT MAKES ATKINS WORK

That leaves us with the third, last, and most (unfairly) maligned mac-ronutrient: fat, which often comes packaged with protein in foods. Okay, I know what you're thinking: "Why can't I just eat no fat or very little fat and burn only my body fat?" There are several reasons this approach won't work:

- Eating adequate fats (at least healthy fats) is essential for life.
- Dietary fats allow your body to absorb the fat-soluble vitamins A, D, E, and K, plus other micronutrients in vegetables.
- Consuming fat stimulates the burning of body fat.
- Without dietary fat, you'd have to rely on carbs and protein for energy, but if you take in more than a certain amount of carbs, you'll remain on a primarily sugar metabolism, and if you rely on too much protein, you won't feel as well.

Bottom line: there's no way to get the calories (energy) you need and to switch to a primarily fat metabolism without dietary fat.

FOUR PHASES, FOUR OBJECTIVES

An all-too-common misconception is that the first phase of Atkins, known as Induction, is the whole programme. That's undoubtedly where many people get the idea that on Atkins you eat only a small amount of carbs and omit major food groups from your diet. Well, nothing could be further from the truth. Just as you don't go directly from reception to year three, or from year six to A-levels, each of the four phases has a distinct purpose. And, just as with your education, each progressively less restrictive phase builds on the prior one as it stakes out new territory.

Okay, so listen to this. Essential to success on Atkins is the process of finding the maximum number of grams of carbs you can consume while continuing to lose weight, keep your appetite under control, and stay alert and energised. This number represents your personal carb balance, which is different for each individual. It also typically increases as you lose weight. To find it, you'll gradually increase both the amount and variety of carbohydrate foods you eat. Learning how to balance your carb intake with continued weight loss is what makes Atkins unique. Then, once you've reached your goal weight, you'll find the maximum number of grams of carbs you can consume while maintaining that weight, staying on top of cravings, and feeling good. This number represents your personal carb tolerance.

In Part II, I'll explain in detail how to approach each phase and offer ways to simplify the programme. There you'll also learn how to move naturally from one phase to the next and finally to embark on your new permanent way of eating. But, for now, let's take a quick snapshot of each of the four phases of the New Atkins Diet.

- **Phase 1: Induction (Kick-Start)**
  How long: A minimum of two weeks, but you may safely follow it for much longer if you have a lot of excess weight to lose or prefer to lose most of your excess pounds relatively quickly, using the Fast Track (pages 85–6). In this case, you'll stay in this phase until you're 7 kg (15 lb) from your goal weight.

Purpose: Shift your body from burning primarily carbs to burning primarily fat, kick-starting weight loss.

Strategy: Significantly drop your daily Net Carb intake to an average of 20 grams of Net Carbs (no less than 18 and no more than 22 grams), the level at which almost anyone begins to burn primarily fat.

- **Phase 2: Ongoing Weight Loss (Balancing)**
  How long: Typically until you're within 4.5 kg (10 lb) of your goal weight, although you can move to Phase 3 sooner if you're willing to slow the pace of weight loss.
  Purpose: Lose most of your excess weight and find your personal carb balance.
  Strategy: Starting at 25 grams of Net Carbs daily, begin to increase overall carb intake in 5-gram increments. This means gradually reintroducing a broader array of carb foods as you step up the Carb Ladder, finding your personal carb balance. It could level off anywhere between 30 and 80 daily grams of Net Carbs or even higher. Your personal number is affected by your age, gender, activity level, hormonal status, and other factors as you continue to lose weight.

- **Phase 3: Pre-Maintenance (Fine-Tuning)**
  How long: Until you've reached your goal weight and maintained it for a month.
  Purpose: Trim your final excess weight, continuing to explore your personal carb balance. Then find your tolerance for carb intake while maintaining your new weight. This phase is a dress rehearsal for Life-time Maintenance.
  Strategy: Gradually increase your daily Net Carb intake in 10-gram (or 5-gram, if you prefer) increments, continuing to reintroduce new carb foods, as long as you continue to slowly lose weight and then to maintain that loss.

- **Phase 4: Lifetime Maintenance**
  How long: Ongoing.
  Purpose: Transition to a permanent way of eating that allows you to maintain your new weight.

Strategy: Remain in control of your weight by adjusting your carb intake if your carb tolerance changes or you regain a few pounds.

WHAT ARE NET CARBS?

You'll use a carb counter to track your daily carbohydrate intake. The downloadable Atkins Carb Counter is available in a printed version and online, as well as a phone app. When counting carbs in the UK/EU the method differs slightly from US labels. On US labels, fibre is included in the total carb content but does not impact your blood sugar, so for US products the Net Carbs are total grams of carbs minus grams of fibre. However, in the UK and EU, fibre is shown separately so there's no need to deduct it. So the 'total carb' amount is what you're counting and not minusing anything out, so it's actually easier to count carbs.

In the case of low-carb foods, sugar alcohols (polyols) are likewise not digested so grams of glycerin, maltitol, mannitol, sorbitol, xylitol and other sugar alcohols are also subtracted from total carbs. This is reflected on the label on low-carb bars and shakes and other foods.

Here's how it works. Say the total grams of carbs listed on a bar's Nutrition Information panel is 10, with 10 grams of fibre and 7 grams of sugar alcohols. The Net Carb count would be 3 grams.

THE CARB LADDER

The Carb Ladder (see page 14) offers a logical progression in which to reintroduce carbohydrate foods as you shed weight. It also makes it easy to move through the first three phases of the New Atkins Diet and then transition to a lifestyle that allows you to maintain your new weight. Even once you've added back certain foods, you'll eat those on the lower rungs most frequently and those on the higher rungs less often. If you have a low carb tolerance, you may not be able to eat some of the foods on the top rungs, or you can have them only rarely. Atkins products are not listed below because they vary in carb impact; most are acceptable in Phase 1, but check the phase coding on the package to be sure.

STEP UP TO WEIGHT LOSS

The illustration entitled Carb Balancing – Steps to Weight Loss, which appears on page 15, shows how the rungs of the Carb Ladder fit within the three weight-loss phases. Important points to understand:

- On the far right, the daily range of Net Carb intake in grams ranges from 20–70, as indicated by the vertical arrow, corresponding to the rungs of the Carb Ladder.
- The ease with which each individual loses weight varies significantly, so the weight-loss numbers merely illustrate that as weight melts away, you'll gradually reintroduce categories of carb foods in a certain order.
- The amount of weight you plan to lose may be more or less than the example shown.
- Likewise, the number of daily grams of Net Carbs you'll reach in Phases 2 and 3 may be greater or smaller.
- The horizontal arrows illustrate when to introduce food groups for both the Fast Track and the Slow and Steady path to weight loss.

Phase 1

Rung 1: Foundation vegetables – leafy greens and other low-carb vegetables

Rung 2: Dairy foods high in fat and low in carbs – cream, soured cream, and most cheeses

Phase 2

Rung 3: Nuts and seeds* (but not chestnuts)

Rung 4: Berries, cherries, and melon (but not watermelon)

Rung 5: Whole milk yoghurt and fresh cheeses such as cottage cheese and ricotta

Rung 6: Legumes, including chickpeas, lentils, and the like

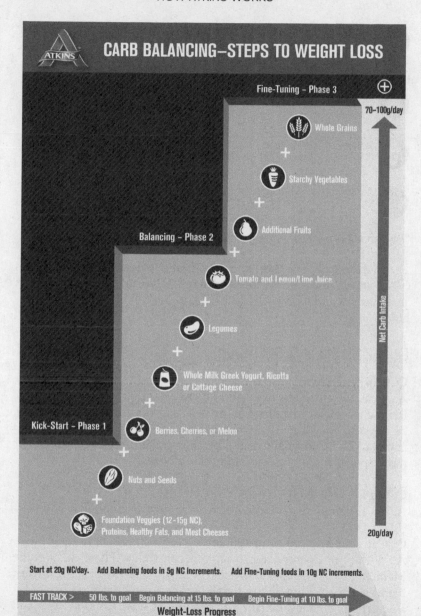

CARB BALANCING—STEPS TO WEIGHT LOSS

Fine-Tuning – Phase 3

70–100g/day

Whole Grains

+

Starchy Vegetables

+

Additional Fruits

+

Balancing – Phase 2

Tomato and Lemon/Lime Juice

+

Legumes

+

Whole Milk Greek Yogurt, Ricotta or Cottage Cheese

+

Kick-Start – Phase 1

Berries, Cherries, or Melon

+

Nuts and Seeds

+

Foundation Veggies (12–15g NC), Proteins, Healthy Fats, and Most Cheeses

Net Carb Intake

20g/day

Start at 20g NC/day.   Add Balancing foods in 5g NC increments.   Add Fine-Tuning foods in 10g NC increments.

FAST TRACK >   50 lbs. to goal   Begin Balancing at 15 lbs. to goal   Begin Fine-Tuning at 10 lbs. to goal

Weight-Loss Progress

SLOW & STEADY > 50 lbs. to goal   Begin Balancing at 40 lbs. to goal   Begin Fine-Tuning at 10 lbs. to goal

Rung 7:   Tomato and vegetable juice "cocktail" (plus more lemon and lime juice)

Phases 3 and 4

 Rung 8:   Other fruits (but not fruit juices or dried fruits)

 Rung 9:   Higher-carb vegetables such as winter squash, carrots, and peas

 Rung 10:   Wholegrains

*You can add nuts and seeds if you stay in Phase 1 beyond two weeks.

For more details, see the list of acceptable Phase 1 foods on pages 30–6, acceptable Phase 2 foods on pages 92–6, and acceptable foods for Phases 3 and 4 on pages 129–134. Phase 3 foods are also acceptable in Phase 4.

FREQUENTLY ASKED QUESTIONS

Q. Can vegetarians do Atkins?
A. Absolutely. It's best to begin at Phase 2 so that you can have nuts, fresh cheeses, and legumes as protein sources from the beginning. See "Atkins for Vegetarians" in Chapter 5. By beginning with 25–30 grams of Net Carbs daily, you'll be able to get sufficient protein. For more specifics, see *The New Atkins for a New You*.

Q. Do I have to eat red meat to do Atkins?
A. No. If you prefer, you can get your protein from poultry and fish.

Q. Can I do Atkins if I'm pregnant?
A. With your doctor's approval, you can follow Phase 4, Lifetime Maintenance. Consume the level of carbs that doesn't stress your blood-sugar level but allows for the proper weight gain necessary for a healthy pregnancy. Be sure to consume at least 1,800 calories and at least 50 to 60 grams of Net Carbs daily. Also eat the recommended

amount of protein, dairy, and fat along with the recommended minimum of foundation vegetables and two servings of fruit a day, plus a
serving of wholegrains if your metabolism allows.

Q. Won't eating lots of fat raise my cholesterol level?
A. No. Research shows that people who comply with Phase 1 of the
Atkins Diet consistently improve their cholesterol profile, especially
their triglycerides. It also raises HDL, the "good" cholesterol. In the
context of a low-carb eating programme, the fat consumed on Atkins
is burned for energy and does not raise the risk for heart disease.

Q. Do I need to count calories on Atkins?
A. Even if you control your carb intake, consuming far too many
calories can interfere with weight loss. It's also possible to consume
too few, which will slow down your metabolism, putting a brake on
weight loss. That said, you're able to eat more (and more satisfying)
food on Atkins than on other weight-loss programmes. The minimum daily calorie range for women is 1,500 to 1,800 calories a day
and 1,800 to 2,200 for men. There's no need to count calories on
Atkins, but if weight loss stalls, do a calorie reality check for a few
days.

Q. Is there a connection between stress and weight loss? How about
sleep?
A. Both stress and lack of sleep can interfere with weight loss. High
levels of the stress hormone cortisol stimulate the release of the fat-
storing hormone insulin. Yoga, stretching, other low-intensity exercise, and meditation can help minimise stress. Likewise, failing to
get at least six hours of sleep a night increases your level of the hunger hormone ghrelin and decreases the level of the hormone leptin,
which makes you feel full. People who sleep more tend to be slimmer than people who sleep less.

Q. Is exercise mandatory?
A. No. Exercise isn't essential to lose weight on Atkins. It is, however, effective to help maintain a healthy weight and to potentially
break a stall. Combining regular activity with dietary changes has
many health benefits and helps elevate mood. Unless you're already

engaged in a regular fitness programme, it's advisable to wait until you're feeling comfortable with your new eating habits before embarking on a new exercise regime. If you've already achieved a certain fitness level, feel free to continue your exercise routine.

Q. Can my overweight child do Atkins?
A. It's important to understand that even a heavy youngster is still growing. No one under the age of 12 should be put on any weight-loss diet before consulting your GP. Meanwhile, weaning your kid off sugar is the single most important thing you can do. If your family starts eating a wholefoods diet, your child will probably lose weight.

In the next chapter, you'll learn how to prepare your kitchen before you embark on Atkins, and take care of some other details so you can hit the ground running. And yes, it's time to take that dreaded "before" photo. Believe me, you'll be glad you did a few months from now, when you greet that slim new you in the mirror every morning! But first meet Tori B., who lost 45 kg (100 lb) on Atkins, giving her the courage to initiate many other changes in her life.

A SLIM AND HEALTHY ROLE MODEL FOR HER DAUGHTERS

VITAL STATS

Daily Net Carb intake:
  20–40 grams
Age: 37
Height: 167 cm (5 ft 6 in)

Before weight: 107 kg
  (16 st 9 lb)
After weight: 62 kg (9 st 7 lb)
Lost: 45 kg (100 lb)

Tori B. was the grand prize winner of the 2012 Atkins weight-loss competition. It was a big deal for her to fly from her home in South Barre, Vermont, to Los Angeles with her husband on their prize holiday, where she met with Atkins spokesperson Sharon Osbourne. "I used to be scared of everything before I lost weight, including flying. I'd even worry that I couldn't fit in a roller coaster seat," she recalls. But after losing 45 kg

(100 lb) on Atkins, Tori welcomes challenges and savours every day of her new life, as she explains.

I was never a heavy kid but, after I hit puberty, my weight became a problem. You name it, I tried it, but I would always regain the lost pounds. After the birth of Grace, who is now 9 years old, I had a miscarriage. I wanted to do everything I could to ensure a healthy infant the next time. Around this time my husband got a new job, and I was in a position to stop working and devote myself to motherhood and getting slim and healthy.

Why did I choose Atkins? I sat down and thought about what I was eating and wrote it all down. It was all carbs, so obviously that was my issue. Also, I wasn't very active before I started Atkins. I was on a high the first day and had already lost 1 kg (2 lb) by the second day. Two weeks after I started Atkins my energy returned and I felt better emotionally.

I started walking 5 km (3 miles) every day through Vermont's beautiful cou tryside. I lost weight consistently, which motivated me to continue. Within three months I'd lost 23 kg (50 lb). My husband was very supportive, which also helped. He lost weight without even trying just by eating what I was eating!

At this point I realised I was pregnant again, so I switched to a modified version of Induction with my doctor's approval. Grace now has a 5-year-old sister, Anne. After her birth I wanted to achieve a total loss of 45 kg (100 lb) so I could be a healthy role model for the girls. Of course, I also wanted this for myself. I knew I needed to take care of me so that I'd be there for them for a good long time. With the well-balanced array of foods you eat on Atkins and exercise, those last pounds melted away. There aren't enough words to describe how incredible I feel. Atkins empowered me to live life more fully and try new things, like Zumba. I've never been so healthy and so in shape. And it's not just me. The whole family skis, snowshoes, and bicycles together.

I hold myself accountable for everything I eat. I weigh myself every day. I figure if I'm going to do it, I'm going to do it right.

I never feel hungry as long as I stay away from starches. Mornings are crazy with two kids to get out the door, so I have an Atkins Day Break Chocolate Hazelnut Bar. I call it my "get-up-and-go bar". Then around 9.30 or 10am I'll have a real breakfast.

My children don't know the unhealthy mum and don't recognise the old me in pictures. More than ever I feel that little girls need healthy guidance about body image and to be shown by example. And though I started out just wanting to be a role model for our daughters, now my transformation has also influenced my extended family. There's a history of heart disease, high cholesterol and hypertension, so they were worried about my eating red meat, eggs, and cheese. Now they see that I also eat lots of vegetables and that foods like doughnuts, biscuits and sugary cereals never make it into my house.

Winning the contest was amazing, as was meeting Sharon Osbourne. The old Tori never could have put her story out there by entering the Atkins competition. The Atkins lifestyle is truly a blessing. If you can find it within yourself to take the journey and follow it through, you'll see how fantastic this lifestyle is. If you eat the right foods and exercise, this way of being will change your outlook on life. I couldn't be prouder of where I am today compared to where I started.

MAKE IT EASY

I literally write down everything I eat, even a little piece of Cheddar cheese, in a notebook. That way if I gain a pound or two it's easy to see what caused it. —TB

CHAPTER 2

PREPARE TO SUCCEED

Now that you know that Atkins is an easy and great-tasting way to lose weight, as well as the basics of how it works, let's get going! Once you finish this chapter, you'll be able to start the New Atkins Diet and begin the exciting process of changing your metabolism, taking control of your appetite, improving your appearance, and boosting your self-image! Let's deal with a few practical matters first, so that you get off on the right foot from the start.

Clearly, having the right food in the fridge, freezer, and store cupboard is essential, so this chapter includes a list of the kinds of foods you can eat in Phase 1. You'll be amazed and delighted at how many tasty and satisfying choices there are. I'll also introduce you to some exciting new digital tools that will make it easier than ever to slim down on Atkins, and remind you about some of the time-honoured aids to help you set your goal weight, track your progress, and achieve your goal.

DOCUMENT THE "BEFORE" YOU

Everyone loves to look at "before and after" photos, particularly when they reveal an almost unbelievable transformation. You're probably already envisioning the sleeker, sexier, and more energised new you. Hold that image – it's key to making your dream a reality. But let's deal with the current you first. Ask a friend to capture a full-length photograph of you, or set it up yourself by using the delayed shutter action feature on your camera. Paste the photo into your journal (or attach it to your online journal or save it on your mobile phone; we'll get to that in a moment), noting the date. Or place it where you'll see it several times a day, such as on the refrigerator door or bathroom mirror.

Why is this photo so important? Initially it serves as an ongoing reminder of what you want to change about yourself. As time goes by, it becomes proof positive of your progress. And when you find yourself tempted by a high-carb treat, that "before" photo can help you resolve not to let a moment on your lips become a lifetime on your hips. Believe me, the day will come when you'll find it hard to believe that you were the person in that photo – and what a thrill that will be!

WEIGH IN AND MEASURE UP

Just as a "before" photo serves as a baseline, weighing yourself before you begin Atkins allows you to track your progress. Although this is hardly your favourite activity at the moment, I promise you that as the weeks go by, you'll find it an increasingly pleasurable one. You can be nude, in your underwear, or clothed, but do take off your shoes. Ideally, weigh in after you've emptied your bladder and before breakfast. Also measure your chest, waist, hips, and thighs. Enter those baseline numbers in your journal to gauge your progress going forward. Thereafter, weigh yourself once a week at the same time, using the same set of scales, if possible, and measure yourself. Why just once a week? It's natural for your weight to fluctuate from day to day and even within a day, depending on your body's natural processes. A weekly weigh-in is a better indicator of how much weight you've lost. Also, checking daily could discourage you when progress is slow or you appear to have regained a pound or two. It's perfectly natural not to lose weight every day no matter how diligently you follow the Atkins programme. You may lose nothing for four days, then appear to suddenly lose 1 kg (2 lb). Weighing weekly minimises such natural variations. If you feel compelled to get on the scales every day, weight averaging is another option (see pages 39).

SET YOUR GOAL WEIGHT

Don't obsess about a particular number if you don't already have one in mind. Just set a reasonable and realistic goal to aim for. You can always adjust your goal weight as you move through the programme. The real objective is to make your goal tangible so that you can visualise the new you waiting to emerge. Once you come up with a number you're comfortable with, enter it in your journal.

If you have a significant amount of weight to lose, you may choose to establish some incremental goals and peg them to specific dates. You'll still keep your ultimate goal at the front of your mind, of course, but every time you shed another 5–7 kg (10–15 lb), you'll have reason to celebrate rather than feel overwhelmed by the longer road ahead. This is exactly what Natalie (page 164) did. Her objective to lose 118 kg (260 lb) was so daunting that she set incremental goals. "That way, every time I lost 2.2 kg (5 lb)," she says, "I felt good about myself, and that kept me going."

TO GET RESULTS, GET SPECIFIC

The more quantifiable a goal, the more likely you are to achieve it. No matter how optimistic you are, "I just want to slim down fast" or "I want to lose oodles of pounds" won't work. Naming your goal weight and adding other specific details, such as why you want to achieve that weight and the time frame in which to do so, makes the goal more tangible and reminds you of why you're going to stay the course.

For example:

- "I want to get to 63 kg (140 lb) so that I can feel comfortable in a swimming costume by the time the pool opens."
- "My goal is to lose 9 kg (20 lb) by our wedding anniversary so that I can wear that fabulous dress I got on our honeymoon."
- "My daughter is getting married a year from now, and I'm going to be 32 kg (70 lb) slimmer so I can fit into my old dinner jacket when I give her away at the altar."

Come up with your own reasons and enter them in your journal.

STAY REAL

When setting your goal weight, make it achievable. Don't set yourself up for disappointment, or worse, by being overly ambitious. Say you've gained 23 kg (50 lb) and had two children since you left school 25 years ago. You've just agreed to go to your reunion in three months' time. It's unlikely that you can meet a goal of losing that 23 kg (50 lb) in that time frame. Even with a realistic timeline, understand that you may not be able to achieve the same weight at age 43 that you were at 18 years old. Your metabolism has almost certainly changed over the years. A better approach would be to set a more reasonable goal, such as 5 kg (10 lb) heavier than your school-leaving weight. When you reach that weight, celebrate your success, and consider resetting your goal.

ASSEMBLE YOUR ATKINS TOOL KIT

You need just four items to track your weight, measurements, and carb intake. Having these to hand from the beginning will allow you to track and record your progress.

1. *A set of scales.* No need for any fancy bells and whistles. If necessary, weigh in at your office, gym, or pharmacy.
2. *A fabric measuring tape.* Inches and centimetres are as important as pounds and kilos in tracking your progress and may show changes before weight loss registers.
3. *Atkins Carb Counter and Acceptable Foods List.* Download this handy, pocket-sized list (referred to as the Atkins Carb Counter from here on) of acceptable foods for each phase of Atkins, along with the Carb counts for hundreds of wholefoods, Atkins products, and meals and beverages at popular restaurant chains. You'll find it at atkins.com. This information is also available as an app for your phone or tablet.
4. *A journal or notebook.* You'll be entering your weight and measurements weekly and recording your food intake and Net Carb count daily. Research consistently shows that people who keep a journal lose more weight than those who don't. *The New Atkins for a New You Workbook* is specially designed to comply with the Atkins programme, but a simple notebook can do

the trick as well. Or use the Atkins online tools. Remember, these numbers are for your eyes only. Pretty soon you'll see the weights and measurements numbers going down, down, down. Also, feel free to record your thoughts and feelings about your weight-loss journey.

EXPLORE THE ATKINS ONLINE RESOURCES AND MOBILE APP

In addition to the items in your basic tool kit, go to atkins.com to access these resources:

- A carb counter that lists hundreds of foods and tracks your daily carb intake
- Additional meal planners, giving a 2-week meal plan for each phase
- Online trackers for your weight and BMI
- A BMI calculator
- The Atkins database of hundreds of recipes, with customised shopping lists for each recipe

If you have a smartphone, download the free Atkins app. These features make it easier than ever to follow the programme, especially when you're on the move:

- *Carb Calculator*. Nutritional information on hundreds of items in the supermarket, hundreds of Atkins recipes, and Atkins products.
- *Progress Tracker*. Helps you to monitor your progress by tallying your daily Net Carb intake and weight, and calculating how close you are to your goal weight.
- *Phase Overview*. A list of the acceptable foods for each of the four Atkins phases.
- *Daily Food Plan*. Both recommended and customisable plans (based on your carb intake and food preferences) for each phase.
- *Recipe Database*. Search hundreds of recipes by phase or key ingredients.

BUILD YOUR ATKINS LIBRARY

Want to learn more? If you're interested in delving deeper into why Atkins works and the research that validates this approach, check out *The New Atkins for a New You*. And if cooking is your thing, you'll find 200 recipes for delectable low-carb meals that you can put together in 30 minutes or less in *The New Atkins for a New You Cookbook*. Both print and electronic versions are available at book shops everywhere, as well as on Amazon and other similar sites.

MAKE YOUR KITCHEN ATKINS-FRIENDLY

Unless you have superior self-control, it's best to remove temptation in the form of high-carb foods, at least for the first few weeks on Atkins. Once you've switched over to burning primarily fat for energy, your desire for crisps, biscuits, doughnuts, sweets, and so forth will be suppressed. Hard to believe, but true! There are also plenty of tasty low-carb substitutes for most of them. But for now, removing problematic foods (or setting them apart from other foods) is the best strategy, perhaps by giving them to a friend, a neighbour, or even a food bank. That means breakfast cereals, bread, pasta, sweets, and anything else made with refined grains and/or sugar. But out with the old unacceptable foods is only half the strategy; the other half is having the right foods in the house.

SHOP FOR SUCCESS

The last thing you want is to find that there's nothing in the house you can eat on your first day on Atkins. The components of a low-carb meal aren't unusual or exotic. With the very occasional exception, everything you need is available at your supermarket. Speciality items such as starch-free thickener for making low-carb gravy can be easily ordered online. To make things super easy for you, we've come up with meal plans for your first two weeks on Atkins (see pages 54–5 and 76–7), along with shopping lists, so that you'll have everything you need to hit the ground running. No later than the day before you start Atkins, photocopy the first shopping list and get yourself to the shops.

WHAT TO LOOK FOR ON A FOOD LABEL

Being able to understand the data on a food label will help you steer clear of high-carb or otherwise problematic ingredients. Food manufacturers don't make it easy for you, so read carefully. There are two parts to a label, both of which contain vital information:

- The Nutrition Information panel lists the serving size, number of calories in a serving – 350 ml (12 fl oz) can of fizzy drink or another beverage may actually be two or more servings – and the amounts of macronutrients, including carbs, fat, and protein, in grams and sometimes as a percentage of the recommended Daily Allowance. Ditto for certain micronutrients, including fibre and some vitamins. Remember, on UK/EU labels, there is no need to subtract grams of fibre from total grams of carbs to get the Net Carbs. Simply count the total carbs to get the right amount.
- The ingredient list includes everything in the product, in order of volume. Here's where you might find one of the umpteen aliases for sugar (see page 58) or other unacceptable ingredients such as hydrogenated vegetable oil or trans fats.

Nutrition Facts

Serving Size 2 Tbsp (32g)

Amount per Serving

Calories 190
Calories from Fat 130

	% Daily Value*
Total Fat 16g	24%
Saturated Fat 2.5g	13%
Trans Fat 0g	
Cholesterol 0mg	0%
Sodium 140mg	6%
Total Carbohydrate 8g	3%
Dietary Fiber 2g	9%
Sugars 3g	
Protein 7g	

Vitamin E	10%	Iron	4%
Niacin	20%	Riboflavin	2%

Not a significant source of vitamin A, vitamin C and calcium.

*Percent Daily Values are based on a 2,000 calorie diet.

Ingredients:
MADE FROM ROASTED PEANUTS AND SUGAR. CONTAINS 2% OR LESS OF MOLASSES, FULLY HYDROGENATED VEGETABLE OILS (RAPESEED AND SOYBEAN), MONO AND DIGLYCERIDES, SALT.

Kosher Information:
Ⓤ

HOW TO IDENTIFY ADDED SUGAR

Packaged food labels don't make it easy for you to judge whether the sugar in a product is added or naturally occurring. You can distinguish whether a product has naturally occurring sugar, added sugar, or both. But when it contains both kinds, there's no way to know how much of each.

1. The Nutrition Information panel lists the number of grams of sugar in a serving. In the case of a 120 g (4 oz) container of a particular berry yoghurt, made with semi-skimmed milk, the label lists 27 grams of sugar.

2. When we look at the list of ingredients, the first ingredient is semi-skimmed milk, which contains naturally occurring sugars. But, tellingly, fructose syrup and sugar are listed before blueberries, which are followed by high-fructose corn syrup. Ingredients are listed in order of highest content, meaning there are more of these two added sugars than a key fruit.

3. So we've learned that there are lots of added sugars in this supposedly nutritious food, but we have no way to quantify the added sugar as opposed to the naturally occurring sugar.

This single example makes a strong case for having the Nutrition Information panel distinguish between the two kinds of sugar.

THE SCOOP ON SUGAR: A GLOSSARY OF SWEETS

The terminology used to describe the absence or presence of sugar can be confusing, especially when you're new to low-carb eating and trying to make smart buying decisions. A few definitions should cut through the doublespeak.

- *Added sugar* is not integral to the product. An apple comes by sugar naturally in the form of fructose, but when that fructose is used in a biscuit, for example, it constitutes added sugar. You want to avoid all added sugars, sometimes referred to as "hidden sugars".
- *Low (or reduced) sugar* suggests that there is less added sugar than is typical in a product, but it still contains added sugar. Avoid such products.
- *Natural sugar* is a term likely to appear on the labels of so-called health food products. Whether honey, molasses, or agave syrup, natural sugar is still sugar.
- *No added sugar* means that a food contains only integral sugars. Examples would be any raw or cooked vegetable, fruit, wholegrains, or unflavoured dairy products.
- *No table sugar* merely means that a food contains no sucrose, but very likely it contains other natural or processed sugars. Again, sugar is sugar.
- *Sugar-free* asserts that a food contains no natural sugars, whether integral or added. Only oils, fats, and a few types of meat and other protein sources are naturally sugar-free.

ACCEPTABLE PHASE 1 FOODS

Now let's preview the delectable foods you get to eat in Phase 1 (Kick-Start), along with a few to avoid. Rather than overwhelm you with the hundreds of vegetables and dozens of cheeses, for example, I've listed just a few common ones here. For more extensive lists, and for serving sizes complete with grams of Carbs, download the Atkins Carb Counter, which includes Acceptable Foods Lists at atkins.com or use the mobile app.

PROTEIN FOODS

- All fish, whether fresh, frozen, tinned, or vacuum packed . . . except:
  - Anything deep-fried, stuffed, breaded, battered, or coated in flour
  - Pickled or creamed herring that contains added sugar
- Shellfish, including crab, oysters, prawns, and clams . . . except:
  - Anything deep-fried, breaded, battered, or coated in flour
  - And limit oysters and mussels, which contain carbs
- All poultry . . . except:
  - Chicken nuggets, breaded portions, or anything that has been deep-fried, stuffed, breaded, battered, or coated in flour
  - Chicken or turkey sausages that contain fillers or other high-carb ingredients
- Beef, lamb, pork, and all other meats, including game . . . except:
  - Products that contain fillers and/or added sugar, including hot dogs*, sausages*, salami*, and mortadella*
  - Meatballs, meatloaf, minced beef steak, and anything stuffed with bread crumbs
- Eggs prepared in any fashion (each egg contains 0.6 grams of Net Carbs)

*We recommend nitrate-free products whenever possible.

OILS AND FATS

No need to count carbs here. Oils are one of the few foods that contain just a single macronutrient: fat! A typical serving size is 1 tablespoon.

Choose from among:

- Butter, hard or whipped
- Rapeseed oil
- Coconut oil
- Flaxseed oil
- Grapeseed oil
- Mayonnaise†
- Olive oil
- High-oleic safflower oil
- Sesame oil

† Mayonnaise contains a minute amount of carbs. Choose a brand made with rapeseed oil or high-oleic safflower oil, not soybean or vegetable oil, whenever possible.

CHEESE

Most cheeses contain less than 1 gram of Net Carbs per 30 g (1 oz) of cheese and are fine in this phase, with the exception of cottage cheese and ricotta, which you'll be able to add in Phase 2. Don't exceed 115 g (4 oz) a day, the equivalent of four individually wrapped slices or cubes the size of large dice. A tablespoon or two of any grated cheese contains a negligible amount of carbs. Select whole-milk products. Avoid low-fat cheeses, "diet" cheese, "cheese products" and whey cheese and any cheese flavoured with fruit. Common cheeses are listed below. Consult the Atkins Carb Counter for a more extensive list.

- Blue cheese
- Brie
- Cheddar
- Cream cheese
- Emmental
- Feta
- Goat's cheese
- Gouda

- Mozzarella, made with whole milk
- Parmesan
- Romano

ADDITIONAL DAIRY PRODUCTS AND DAIRY SUBSTITUTES

Feel free to use up to 45ml (1½ fl oz) daily or a total of 2–3 table-spoons soured cream, unsweetened whipping cream, or single cream in your coffee or tea. Most so-called non-dairy substitutes for milk or cream are full of sugar or high-fructose corn syrup, and all too often they contain unhealthy trans fats as well. However, we've found a few unsweetened "creamers" for coffee and tea without these problematic ingredients. A tablespoon of each contains no more than 1 gram of Carbs. See the Atkins Carb Counter for more details.

- Double cream, liquid or whipped
- Single cream
- Soured cream, full-fat
- Also Alpro Unsweetened soya milk

Milk is off the menu for the time being, but you can have a cup of several different milk substitutes at 1–2 grams of Net Carbs. All should be plain (unflavoured) and sugar-free:

- Almond milk
- Coconut milk beverage (not tinned coconut milk)
- Soya milk

FOUNDATION VEGETABLES

There is a wealth of vegetables acceptable in Phase 1, but we'll keep the list to a minimum for simplicity's sake. They include salad leaves and other salad ingredients, as well as vegetables that are typically cooked. Your daily minimum of 12–15 grams of Net Carbs translates into about 175 g (6 oz) of salad leaves and 200–300 g (7–11 oz) cooked vegetables. (If you're not sure how to get all those vegetables in, see the meal plans in the following chapters.) Try to have both types each day, but have more salad leaves and cut back on cooked ones if you prefer. Frozen vegetables are fine.

SALAD LEAVES About 30 g (1 oz) of each of the following raw salad leaves comes in at less than 1 gram of Net Carbs:

- Cabbage
- Endive
- Lettuce, all types
- Rocket
- Spinach
- Sprouts, all kinds
- Watercress

OTHER SALAD VEGETABLES These are usually slightly higher in carbs. Consult the Atkins Carb Counter for more details on serving sizes and carb counts.

- Avocados, Hass
- Bamboo shoots, tinned
- Celery
- Cucumber
- Mushrooms
- Olives, black or green
- Onions
- Gherkins, dill or sour
- Radishes, Daikon
- Spring onions
- Sweet peppers, any colour
- Tomatoes

VEGETABLES (TYPICALLY COOKED) About 60 g (2 oz) of the following cooked vegetables contain no more than 3 grams of Net Carbs. (Be sure to measure them after cooking rather than before.) Those with an asterisk have considerably less.

- Asparagus
- Aubergine
- Beans, French, bobby, broad, green
- Broccoli
- Cauliflower*
- Chard*
- Courgettes and other summer squash*

- Kale
- Mushrooms
- Okra
- Sauerkraut*
- Spinach*
- Squash, spaghetti
- Turnips

BEVERAGES

Water can be bottled, filtered, mineral, spring, sparkling, or from the tap. Jazz up H_2O with a couple of tablespoons of lemon and/or lime juice, if you wish. Most vitamin waters are full of added sugar (see "The Scoop on Sugar: Multiple Aliases" on page 58), but a few brands with acceptable sweeteners have zero grams of carbs. Ditto for tins or bottles of iced teas, but always check the Nutrition Information panel to uncover any added sugar. You can also have hot chocolate mixes sweetened with non-caloric sweeteners and mixed with water (and a splash of cream) instead of milk.

- Coffee (caffeinated or decaffeinated, hot or iced) and espresso
- Tea (caffeinated or decaffeinated); sugar-free iced tea (brewed, bottled, or tinned)
- Herbal teas and infusions without added sugar
- Soda water
- Diet fizzy drinks sweetened with non-caloric sweeteners, such as Diet Coke, Pepsi Max and Diet Lemonade
- Sugar-free tonic water

CONDIMENTS AND SEASONINGS

Such flavour enhancers add zest to meals. All fresh herbs are acceptable in this phase and contain virtually no carbs. So are small amounts of dried herbs, including basil, bay leaves, chives, coriander, cumin, oregano, rosemary, thyme, and others, plus salt and pepper. Most spices and spice mixes such as chilli powder and curry powder are fine, but avoid spice mixes that contain added sugar. Again, this list gives just a small taste of the condiments and seasonings you can use in Induction.

- Bacon bits
- Celery salt
- Chilli peppers
- Garlic
- Ginger root
- Italian seasoning
- Lemon or orange peel, grated
- Paprika
- Red chilli flakes
- Mustard (without added sugar)
- Poultry seasoning

SAUCES

This category is a bit of a minefield. While one brand of, say, barbecue sauce may be made without sugar, another may be swimming in it. Check the Nutrition Information panel carefully for added sugars as well as flour and other starches.

- Barbecue sauce
- Cocktail/seafood sauce
- Enchilada sauce
- Garlic sauce
- Horseradish sauce
- Ketchup
- Pasta or pizza sauce
- Pesto sauce
- Salsa
- Sofrito
- Soya sauce or tamari
- Steak sauce and marinade
- Tabasco or other hot sauce
- Taco sauce, green or red
- Thai fish sauce

Tomato sauce, tinned or stewed tomatoes, tomato purée, and tomato paste are all acceptable in Induction, as long as they contain no added sugar.

SALAD DRESSINGS

Any prepared salad dressing without added sugar and no more than 3 grams of Net Carbs per serving (1–2 tablespoons) is acceptable. A better lower-carb option is to make your own vinaigrette with olive oil plus either vinegar, lemon juice, or lime juice.

- Blue cheese dressing
- Caesar salad dressing
- Italian dressing
- Ranch dressing
- Vinaigrette

You can also have up to 2 tablespoons lemon or lime juice a day.

NON-CALORIC SWEETENERS

Count each packet as 1 gram of Net Carbs, and consume no more than three per day. Although the sweeteners themselves contain no carbs, the powdered agent that keeps them from clumping has a small amount.

- Splenda or Sweetex (sucralose)
- Truvia (a natural product made from stevia)
- Canderel (a blend of aspartame, acesulfame-K, sucralose and stevia)
- Sweet'n Low (saccharin)
- Xylitol (available in health food shops and some supermarkets).

ATKINS LOW-CARB PRODUCTS

All Atkins products are coded for appropriate phases.

- All Atkins Advantage Bars
- All Atkins Ready-to-Drink Shakes
- All Atkins Day Break Bars
- All Atkins shake mixes
- Atkins Advantage Wheat & Rye Crackers
- Atkins Day Break Bread mix

You can also eat certain other low-carb foods so long as they contain no more than 3 grams of Net Carbs per serving.

SUPERMARKET TIPS

What if cooking from scratch is not your thing or you rarely have the time? Not to worry. This book is all about making Atkins easy. In addition to the delectable Atkins meals, some of which are suitable for breakfast and others for lunch or dinner, and other products, consider these options:

- Scour the frozen-foods section for products such as burgers in single servings, chicken breasts, and lots of different vegetables. Some come in their own steaming bags that you can puncture and pop in the microwave oven. No pans to wash!
- Look in the same section for fish portions (the unbreaded kind), scallops, and prawns for super-quick meals.
- Visit the deli section for pre-cooked roast or grilled chicken and turkey that comes in chunks or slices. They're great for tossing together a stir-fry, a main-dish salad, or another no cook or easy-cook meal in no time.

We'll explore these options in greater detail, along with lots more ideas, in Chapter 9.

THE BEST TIME TO START ATKINS

No matter how eager you are to start paring pounds, starting today or tomorrow might not be the best idea. Why wait? If you work outside the home, you might be better off waiting for the weekend, when you have more control of your time and when and what you eat. Or spend the weekend getting ready and turn a new page on Monday morning. You also don't want any added stress occurring simultaneously. So if it's exam week, crunch time at the office, or the first week of a new job, or if your child is sick with the flu, hold off. Likewise, if you're leaving on holiday or it's the festive season when temptation is everywhere, you may want to wait until you can focus on your new way of eating.

That said; don't fall into the trap of always finding an excuse to put off starting until tomorrow or next week. There will always be social and work situations to navigate and temptation wherever you turn. Pick a date and stick to it. You'll be proud of your resolve. Get used to that feeling!

DISCUSS MEDICATIONS WITH YOUR DOCTOR

If you're taking certain prescription drugs, check with your GP before starting Atkins. Insulin, some anti-depressants, steroids, and beta-blockers can interfere with weight loss. He or she may be able to change the dosage or substitute another drug. If you're taking diuretic medications for high blood pressure, losing water weight and then fat may necessitate a reduced dosage. Check your blood pressure regularly and report any change immediately. Finally, your blood-sugar levels will begin to self-regulate on Atkins, so if you're taking insulin, you'll have to reduce your dosage to avoid your blood sugar dropping too low. Test your blood-sugar levels regularly and work closely with your GP.

FREQUENTLY ASKED QUESTIONS

Q. How do I incorporate Atkins products into my eating plan?
A. Atkins products can make all the difference in being able to stay with the programme regardless of where you are at mealtime or snack time. But convenience foods shouldn't replace foundation vegetables and other wholefoods. Make sure to consume at least 12 and preferably 15 of your allotted 20 daily Net Carb grams in the form of foundation vegetables.

Q. Do I have to take vitamin supplements on Atkins?
A. You'll be eating foods full of vitamins, minerals, and antioxidants, but it's still difficult to ensure you're getting all the nutrients you need on a daily basis, so it is just a good insurance policy to take a few supplements. In addition to a daily multivitamin-mineral supplement (without iron unless you're anaemic), I advise taking additional vitamin D and omega-3 fatty acids (unless you're having two or more servings of fatty fish a week). Significant weight loss reduces your stores of omega-3s. Your body makes vitamin D after exposure to sunlight, but levels can diminish in winter or during overcast periods.

Q. What is weight averaging?

A. Your weight naturally fluctuates from day to day, which is why I recommend weighing in once a week. If you must weigh yourself daily, add that number to those from the two previous days, then divide by three to get your average weight. You can even do this on your mobile phone. A running three-day average gives you a better sense of your progress than your weight on any single day.

Q. Which sugar substitutes are suitable for beverages and which for cooking?

A. Packets, tablets and liquid dispensers are handy for sweetening beverages. The granular forms of sucralose and xylitol sold in a bag or box can be used for cooking.

• • •

Now let's move on to Part II, "It's Easy to Become the New You", where we'll examine each of the four phases of the Atkins Diet, starting with Phase 1, which kick-starts weight loss, so you can see results quickly! But first, take a few minutes to be inspired by Charity W., who lost 61 kg (135 lb) on Atkins, enduring two extended periods when the scale wouldn't budge. In her determination to reach her goal, Charity would begin each day repeating "I can do this". And so she did.

THE SECOND TIME'S A CINCH

VITAL STATS

Daily Net Carb intake: 20–50 grams

Age: 37

Height: 162 cm (5 ft 4 in)

Before weight: 128 kg (20 st 3 lb)

After weight: 67 kg (10 st 7 lb)

Lost: 61 kg (135 lb)

Charity W. knew that Atkins works. She'd lost 18 kg (40 lb) in three months on the programme before her 2004 wedding, but after the honeymoon she returned to her old ways, eating lots of pasta and bread, plus "tons of sugar". The Minneapolis, Minnesota resident also loves to bake. So back came the weight and with it came health issues. Charity takes it from here.

In 2010 I visited my in-laws, when photos of the whole family were taken. When the pictures arrived I was very unhappy with them. Was I really that big? I had heard that Atkins had changed, placing more emphasis on vegetables. I read *The New Atkins for a New You*, and I thought, "I can do that, and I can do it for the rest of my life." The first month was the hardest. I had headaches, but drinking broth helped, and by the second week they were gone. Every day when I woke up I would say, "I can do it!" I even wrote these words on my bathroom mirror so they were just about the first thing I saw each morning. By the end of the month, I'd lost 7 kg (15 lb).

After two weeks on Induction, I added nuts. After 12 weeks I stalled at 118 kg (18 st 7 lb) and realised I was overdoing the cheese, so I cut back to 30 g (1 oz) a day. Still the number on the scales wouldn't budge. I was so disheartened that I went to the Atkins Community for help. The advice and encouragement I got were terrific. I stuck with protein, fat, vegetables, and nuts. That did the trick. In one week my body played catch-up, dropping 1.8 kg (4 lb). After six months in Phase 1, I moved to Phase 2, adding berries and yoghurt. I found the berries were causing cravings, so I knocked them out. Within six months I'd lost 25 kg (55 lb), and 11 months after starting I hit the big number: 45 kg (100 lb) gone. Until this point, I hadn't done any exercise. I hit another plateau during the holidays, and started working out. Nonetheless, I stayed at 84 kg (13 st 2 lb) for eight endless weeks. But I stayed with Atkins and the workouts. When I finally hit my goal of 67 kg (10 st 7 lb) after about 16 months, it was one of the happiest days of my life. I did it! Just like I knew I could.

I still love to bake, but I've made some big changes. Instead of wheat flour, I now use almond and coconut flours, plus flaxseed meal for tortillas. My favourite sweeteners are stevia and sugar alcohols, but I use as little as possible. Spices are very important for low-carb baking. I love to try new recipes and have found some great ones on the Atkins website.

I'm very careful about portions. I'll put one or two biscuits in a freezer bag and have only that much for a snack. I've also found my carb tolerance allows me to eat berries and even half an apple, but I stay away from rice, potatoes, and any processed food.

Losing weight has changed a lot of other things in my life. I'd had gestational diabetes in both my pregnancies and been plagued with irritable bowel syndrome and acid reflux for years. Both are now gone. I'm at the gym five or six times a week, often for two or three hours at a time, swimming and doing weights and elliptical training. I used to roller-blade when I was younger, and now I'm doing it again. I also spend more time playing with my kids. Life is good. And Atkins helped me get there.

MAKE IT EASY

Here's my recipe for quick egg muffins. Chop up a pre-cooked sausage and place it in a greased muffin tin with grated cheese and finely chopped onion and sweet peppers – sauté the onion and peppers first. Whisk an egg and pour it over the other ingredients. Bake at 180°C (350°F) until set. Make a batch and freeze in individual plastic freezer bags. Defrost the night before or in the microwave. *—CW*

PART II

IT'S EASY TO BECOME THE NEW YOU

CHAPTER 3

YOUR FIRST WEEK ON ATKINS

Now that you understand how the programme works and the kinds of foods you'll be eating, I have a few questions for you.

- Are you ready to have the body you've always dreamed of?
- Are you ready to eat three yummy meals and two satisfying snacks a day, and still shed weight?
- Are you ready to actually get your appetite under control once and for all?
- Are you ready to reinvent yourself?

If your answer to all four questions is yes – and of course it is – congratulations on taking this important first step towards turning your dreams into reality! And welcome to your first week on Atkins. The purpose of the first phase of the programme, known as Induction, is to kick-start weight loss. Although it takes a few days to actually start losing fat pounds – water pounds come off first – you'll almost certainly see real results by the end of the week. Some people lose as much as a half a kilo or a pound a day.

You'll achieve this amazing feat by dropping your carbohydrate intake to a level at which almost anyone starts burning primarily fat for energy after a few days. Then, like magic, those excess pounds begin to vanish. Even if you have just a little weight to lose or you've decided to begin in a later phase of Atkins, understanding how this first phase works gives you a solid grounding in the whole programme. Doing Atkins right from the beginning will bring faster and more

45

impressive results. My job is to make that as easy as possible for you.

In this chapter you'll find a meal plan for Week 1 (see pages 54–5), with a companion shopping list (page 52) incorporating foods suitable for Phase 1 (the first rung on the Carb Ladder – see page 14), as well as more advice on what to eat and how to prepare it. We'll also go into greater detail about why you should be eating certain foods and passing on others. Finally, we'll discuss some small changes that can spell the difference between immediate success and a frustrating delay.

TEN SIMPLE STEPS FOR SUCCESS

Follow these guidelines to get off on the right foot from day one:

1. *Have three meals and two snacks a day.* Never starve yourself or go more than three or four waking hours without eating. If you prefer, have five or even six small meals. You never want to allow yourself to become ravenously hungry. That can open the door to eating whatever's at hand. Not a good idea!

2. *Consume 20 grams of Carbs a day.* Of these, 12–15 grams should be in the form of foundation vegetables (see pages 32–4). It's fine to average 20 grams a day over several days, but don't go below 18 grams or above 22 on a single day. Dropping below 18 probably won't make you lose weight any faster and is unlikely to satisfy your vegetable requirement. Going above 22 grams could interfere with triggering weight loss. Select carb foods from the list of Phase 1 acceptable foods in the previous chapter.

3. *Eat sufficient protein at every meal.* As you now know, protein plays a key role in weight loss and protects lean muscle mass, so you lose only fat.

4. *Don't restrict fats.* Consuming fat is essential to slimming down on Atkins. Fat also heightens the flavour of foods and enables your body to absorb certain vitamins. Always accompany a carb snack with either fat or protein. For example, have cucumber slices with a piece of cheese.

5. *Drink at least eight 240 ml (8 fl oz) portions of water daily.* Two of these can be replaced with coffee or tea. Another two portions

can be replaced with beef, chicken, or vegetable stock (not the low sodium kind).

6. *Avoid dehydration or electrolyte imbalance.* The perfectly normal initial loss of water weight can lead to light-headedness and other symptoms and rob you of energy. These symptoms disappear once you're burning primarily fat, but in the meantime, be sure to consume sufficient salt in the form of salty stock, salt, tamari, or soya sauce. For more, see "Stop Certain Symptoms Before They Start" on page 56.

7. *Watch out for hidden carbs.* Read food labels carefully, particularly on condiments. In restaurants, ask for oil and vinegar to dress your salad, request sauces on the side, and feel free to ask the server what's in a dish.

8. *Use sugar substitutes – in moderation* (see "Non-caloric Sweeteners" on page 36). That means no more than three per day.

9. *Use only Atkins low-carb products.* Most of these have been tested to ensure that their impact on your blood sugar level is minimal. The majority of them are coded for Phase 1.

10. *Eat nothing that isn't on the list of Phase 1 acceptable foods.*

A WEALTH OF CHOICES

From the start, you can eat a wide range of foods, including almost all forms of animal protein, as well as several vegetarian ones. Pick your favourites, select budget-conscious cuts, or have "meatless Mondays", if you wish. Most animal sources contain no carbs, with a few exceptions noted in the Phase 1 acceptable foods list.

Since fat is not a no-no on Atkins, you can stir-fry meats, poultry, fish, and vegetables in oil, serve protein dishes with cream sauces, top vegetables with a pat of butter, and use oil-based dressings on your salad – all without guilt. However, you don't want to go overboard on protein or fat either, as we'll explain. Most of your initial carbs will come from foundation vegetables, but there are also many condiments and beverages you can enjoy. You'll be counting grams of Net Carbs – remember, in the UK/EU, that's total carbs as fibre is shown separately on labels (deduct sugar alcohols in the case of some low-carb foods).

THE RIGHT FATS . . .

Your objective is to consume a wide variety of natural fats with the most health benefits. So which should you be eating – or not?

- Dress salads and vegetables with extra-virgin olive oil; virgin olive oil is fine for cooking.
- Cook with rapeseed oil and most nut oils. Like olives and avocados, these reduce levels of "bad" (LDL) cholesterol and triglycerides. High-oleic safflower oil handles high heat well.
- You can also cook with butter or coconut oil, and top vegetables and other foods with butter.
- Have two to three servings of fish and/or shellfish weekly.
- Snack on olives and avocados, and include them in salads. Nuts and seeds also make great snacks and garnishes once you've been on Atkins for two weeks.
- There's no need to cut the fat off meat or remove the skin from poultry, but you can do so if you prefer.

Avoid:

- Any oil that has been subjected to nutrient-destroying high heat during processing. Instead, look for cold-pressed oils and store them away from heat sources and direct light.
- Trans fats, which are vegetable oils that have been blasted with hydrogen gas to give them a long shelf-life, have been linked to an increased risk of heart disease and other health problems. The words "hydrogenated" or "partially hydrogenated" on the list of ingredients mean that a product contains trans fats. In addition to most shortenings and some margarines, many commercial baked goods contain trans fats.

. . . AND THE RIGHT AMOUNTS

The trick is to consume enough fat to keep your fat-burning engine humming along, but not so much as to create a calorie bomb that may interfere with weight loss. As with protein, the correct intake depends in part on your gender and size. Small women may need less and big guys may need more, but follow these guidelines and you should be fine. You can replace one with another – 30 ml (1 fl oz) of cream, for example, in lieu of an egg. In addition to the fat in your daily servings of fish, shellfish, poultry, and meat, here's a typical day's fat intake:

- 2 or 3 eggs
- 2 tablespoons olive or another oil for dressing salads and cooking
- 1 tablespoon butter
- 30 ml (1 fl oz) cream
- 55 g (2 oz) cheese
- 10 olives and/or ½ Hass avocado
- 55 g (2 oz) seeds or nuts (after first two weeks on Induction)

There's no need to eat only lean cuts of meat and white-meat poultry. Nor must you remove the skin from chicken or turkey or remove the fat from a steak or pork chop. If you prefer to, fine, but if so, replace the fat with other natural fats.

PORTION CONTROL

Overestimating serving sizes is a common mistake people make on any weight-loss programme. Eat too large a serving of any carb food and you'll likely exceed the initial recommended daily 20 grams of Net Carbs. Overly large portions of protein foods can also stall weight loss. If you don't have a set of baking or food scales or don't want to bother with measuring spoons or cups to track your carb and protein intake, take another approach. Use the familiar objects listed below to visualise and estimate various portion sizes of meat or fish, or a normal portion of steamed spinach or sautéed courgettes. (Foods marked with an asterisk will be introduced in later phases.)

FOOD	FAMILIAR OBJECT
115 g (4 oz) meat, poultry, fish, tofu, etc.	Smartphone
175 g (6 oz) meat, poultry, fish, tofu, etc.	Computer mouse
225 g (8 oz) meat, poultry, tofu, etc.	Slim paperback book
30 g (1 oz) hard cheese	Large dice
85 g (3 oz) salad leaves	Rounders ball
85 g (3 oz) cooked vegetables	Billiard ball

55 g (2 oz) cooked legumes*	Egg, large
2 tablespoons nut butter*	Golf ball
55 g (2 oz) cooked grains*	Tennis ball

WHY SO MANY VEGETABLES?

If you came to Atkins thinking it was all about beef and bacon, you may be surprised to find yourself eating more vegetables than you ever did before. Initially, you'll be eating primarily what we call foundation vegetables (FV), those with a lower carb content and often a higher fibre count than starchy vegetables higher up the Carb Ladder. Powerhouses of vitamins, minerals, and disease-combating antioxidants, vegetables are also full of fibre that helps:

- Fill you up, blunting your appetite for higher-carb foods
- Lower cholesterol
- Prevent constipation and maintain GI health.

The water content of vegetables, particularly foundation vegetables, also helps keep you well hydrated and replaces electrolytes dissolved in the fluids being washed from your body as you shed the first water pounds. Steaming is a quick and simple way to cook vegetables, especially if you microwave them. Or steam fresh or frozen vegetables in a steamer basket. You can also stir-fry, sauté, or grill vegetables, but never boil them (unless you're making soup), which destroys nutrients.

MAKE IT EASY

To avoid waste from spoilage if you're not cooking many meals at home, you may be better off buying frozen vegetables and confining your fresh choices to salad vegetables.

WHICH CARBS ARE OFF-LIMITS FOR NOW?

Now that you know what you can eat in the first few weeks on Atkins, let's look at which foods to avoid:

- Fruit (other than rhubarb, which is really a vegetable). Avocados, olives, and tomatoes – all of which are actually fruit – are fine.
- Fruit juice (other than 2 tablespoons lemon and/or lime juice a day).
- Caloric sodas.
- Bread, pasta, muffins, tortillas, crisps, and any other food made with flour or other grain products, with the exception of low-carb products with 3 grams of Net Carbs or less.
- Any foods made with added sugar of any sort, including but not limited to pastries, biscuits, cakes, and sweets. (See "The Scoop on Sugar: Fat Took the Hit for Sugar" on page 9.)
- Alcohol in any form.
- Nuts and seeds, nut and seed butters, and nut flours or meals, with the exception of flax meal and coconut flour. (Nuts and seeds are okay after two weeks on Phase 1.)
- Grains, even wholegrains.
- Kidney beans, chickpeas, lentils, and other pulses.
- Starchy vegetables such as carrots, potatoes, sweet potatoes, and winter squash. Check the Atkins Carb Counter if you're unsure.
- Dairy products other than cream, soured cream, single cream, and aged cheeses. No cow's or goat's milk, yoghurt, cottage cheese, or ricotta for now.
- "Low-fat" foods, which are usually higher in carbs.
- "Diet" products, unless they specifically state "low carbohydrate" and have no more than 3 grams of Net Carbs per serving.
- "Junk food" in any form.
- Products such as chewing gum, breath mints, cough syrups and drops, or liquid vitamins, unless they're sweetened with sorbitol or xylitol. You can have up to three a day of those. Count 1 gram per piece.

You may want to photocopy this list and place it on your refrigerator door.

WEEK-AT-A-GLANCE WEEK 1 MEAL PLAN

To make things as easy as possible, I've prepared a simple meal plan to follow in your first week, along with a shopping list of everything you'll need. You'll be eating protein, foundation vegetables, and acceptable Phase 1 (Kick-Start) dairy products, as illustrated on the first rung of the Carb Ladder (page 14).

Kick-Start – Phase 1

Foundation Vegetables (12–15 g NC),
Proteins, Healthy Fats, and Most Cheeses

Of course, you can modify the meal plan to suit your preferences as long as you stay within the Phase 1 acceptable foods guidelines. For example:

- If you don't eat red meat, simply substitute fish, shellfish, poultry, or tofu for pork, beef, etc.
- If you prefer other foundation vegetables, substitute them with others on the list.
- You can swap one or more items with a recipe from the recipe section (page 211) or the online recipe database.

WEEK 1 SHOPPING LIST

Assuming you follow the meal plan to the letter, this short shopping list enables you to have everything at hand to get a week's worth of meals on the table. If you're not using Atkins products, simply adjust the list. Likewise, if you modify the meal plan, you'll need to make comparable changes to the shopping list.

The meal plan incorporates a number of Atkins bars and shakes. It requires only 24 common ingredients, a number of which you probably already have in your fridge, store cupboards, or freezer, saving you time both shopping and cooking.

WEEK 1

PROTEINS	DAIRY/CHEESE	VEGETABLES	SAUCES/ CONDIMENTS	ATKINS PRODUCTS
Steak or Beef Burgers	Butter	Hass Avocados	Creamy Italian Dressing*	Atkins Bars
Chicken	Cheddar Cheese	Baby Spinach	Mayonnaise* or Tartare Sauce*	Atkins Shakes
Eggs	Mozzarella Cheese	Broccoli	Ranch Dressing*	Atkins Drinks
Ham or Pork Chops			Celery	Vinaigrette*
Tinned Tuna or Fish Fillets		Lettuce/Salad Leaves	Extra-Virgin Olive Oil	
Bacon or Sausages			Onions	
		Sweet Red Peppers		
		Tomatoes		

*Select sauces and condiments without added sugar.

The plan indicates the number of grams of Net Carbs from foundation vegetables, making it easy to ensure that you're getting enough of these nutritious and filling carbohydrate foods. The plan does not include beverages; add grams of Net Carbs in cream, lighteners, or sweeteners in beverages to your daily tally.

If you're creating your own meal plans, be sure to spread your carb intake out across the day to keep your blood sugar on an even keel. Aim for roughly 3–5 grams of Net Carbs at breakfast, 5–7 at lunch, and the same at dinner. Snacks can range from 1 to 3 grams.

A GAME PLAN FOR MEALS AWAY FROM HOME

If you work outside the home, you're likely to eat out at least once a day. So give some thought to how you're going to find low-carb meals and snacks on those occasions. Think about what your typical day looks like now.

- Which meals do you eat at home?
- Which do you bring to work with you?
- Which do you order out?

Atkins Phase 1 (Kick-Start) Meal Plan at 20 g NC/day: Week 1

	MONDAY	TUESDAY	WEDNESDAY	THURSDAY
BREAKFAST	2 eggs 40 g chopped onion 1 tsp olive oil 30 g Cheddar cheese 60 g bacon or sausage Net Carbs: 4.1 g; FV: 3.1 g	Atkins Advantage Chocolate Hazelnut Crunch Bar Net Carbs: 2.9 g; FV: 0 g	2 eggs 60–115 g ham 1 tbsp olive oil 3 tbsp chopped onion ½ small tomato Net Carbs: 4.6 g; FV: 3.5 g	115–175 g steak or beef burger 1 tsp olive oil 90 g chopped red pepper 40 g chopped onion 60 g Cheddar cheese Net Carbs: 6 g; FV: 5.3 g
SNACK	Atkins Day Break Almond Cranberry Bar Net Carbs: 3.9 g; FV: 0 g	1 small tomato 60 g Cheddar cheese Net Carbs: 2.8 g; FV: 2.5 g	Atkins Day Break Cappuccino Nut Bar Net Carbs: 3.5 g; FV: 0 g	1 celery stick 30 g mozzarella cheese Net Carbs: 1.2 g; FV: 1 g
LUNCH	115–175 g ham or pork chop 1 small tomato 30 g baby spinach 2 tbsp vinaigrette* Net Carbs: 4.3 g; FV: 4 g	115–175 g chicken 1 small tomato 55 g mixed lettuce ½ avocado 2 tbsp ranch dressing* Net Carbs: 5.8 g; FV: 5.1 g	115–175 g steak or beef burger 55 g mixed greens ½ avocado 2 tbsp vinaigrette* Net Carbs: 3 g; FV: 2.6 g	Atkins Advantage Chocolate Decadence Bar Net Carbs: 2 g; FV: 0 g
SNACK	Atkins Advantage Café Royal RTD Net Carbs: 1.3 g; FV: 0 g	1 celery stick 60 g Cheddar cheese Net Carbs: 1.7 g; FV: 1 g	1 small tomato 30 g Cheddar cheese Net Carbs: 2.6 g; FV: 2.5 g	1 small tomato 2 tbsp vinaigrette* Net Carbs: 2.9 g; FV: 2.5 g
DINNER	115–175 g tinned tuna or fish fillet 110 g mixed lettuce ½ avocado 2 tbsp vinaigrette* 90 g broccoli 1 tbsp butter Net Carbs: 6 g; FV: 5.6 g	115–175 g steak or beefburger ½ medium pepper ⅓ small onion 1 tbsp olive oil 55 g mixed lettuce 2 tbsp Ranch Dressing* Net Carbs: 6.3 g; FV: 5.5 g	115–175 g chicken 90 g broccoli florets 1 tbsp olive oil 110 g mixed lettuce 2 tbsp Creamy Italian Dressing* Net Carbs: 4.5 g; FV: 4.3 g	115–175 g chicken 60 g baby spinach 45 g sliced pepper 1 small tomato 2 tbsp Ranch Dressing* Net Carbs: 6.5 g; FV: 5.8 g
	Total Net Carbs: 19.6 g Total Net Carbs from FV: 12.7 g	Total Net Carbs: 19.5 g Total Net Carbs from FV: 14.1 g	Total Net Carbs: 18.2 g Total Net Carbs from FV: 12.9 g	Total Net Carbs: 18.6 g Total Net Carbs from FV: 14.6 g

FRIDAY	SATURDAY	SUNDAY
60 g baby spinach 1 tbsp olive oil 1 small tomato 60 g Cheddar cheese	2 eggs 60 g bacon or sausage 1 small tomato	2 eggs 60 g baby spinach 1 tbsp olive oil ½ red pepper 60 g Cheddar cheese
Net Carbs: 6.8 g; FV: 6.8 g	Net Carbs: 4.5 g; FV: 2.5 g	Net Carbs: 6.4 g; FV: 5.3 g
Atkins Day Break Strawberry Yoghurt RTD	Atkins Day Break Strawberry Crisp Bar	1 celery stick 60 g Cheddar cheese
Net Carbs: 3 g; FV: 0 g	Net Carbs: 3 g; FV: 0 g	Net Carbs: 1.7 g; FV: 1 g
115–175 g chicken 100 g mixed lettuce 45 g sliced pepper 2 tbsp Creamy Italian Dressing*	115–175 g tinned tuna or fish fillet 2 tbsp mayonnaise or tartare sauce* 1 celery stick 45 g chopped red pepper 1 small tomato	Atkins Advantage Dark Chocolate Crunch Bar
Net Carbs: 4.8 g; FV: 4.5 g	Net Carbs: 5 g; FV: 5 g	Net Carbs: 3.7 g; FV: 0 g
Atkins Advantage Milk Chocolate RTD	½ avocado 2 tbsp Creamy Italian Dressing*	90 g chopped red pepper 2 tbsp Ranch Dressing*
Net Carbs: 1.3 g; FV: 0 g	Net Carbs: 1.5 g; FV: 1.3 g	Net Carbs: 2.9 g; FV: 2.2 g
115–175 g ham or pork chop 90 g broccoli 1 tbsp butter 55 g mixed lettuce 1 small tomato 2 tbsp Creamy Italian dressing*	115–175 g steak or beef burger 30 g Cheddar cheese 1 small tomato ½ avocado ½ small onion, sliced	175 g chicken 90 g broccoli 1 tbsp olive oil 55 g mixed lettuce ½ avocado 2 tbsp vinaigrette*
Net Carbs: 5.6 g; FV: 5.4 g	Net Carbs: 6.7 g; FV: 6.5 g	Net Carbs: 4.6 g; FV: 4.2 g
Total Net Carbs: 21.5 g Total Net Carbs from FV: 16.8 g	Total Net Carbs: 20.7 g Total Net Carbs from FV: 15.3 g	Total Net Carbs: 19.3 g Total Net Carbs from FV: 12.7 g

- How often do you eat out?
- Do you take coffee breaks or keep snack foods in your desk or locker?
- Do you often find yourself at train stations or airports, or driving in areas devoid of good food choices, or just sitting in traffic?

Then think about what you actually eat at those times. If you typically grab a bagel on the way to work, eat lunch – usually a sandwich – out, and often order pizza for dinner on week nights, just stocking your kitchen with Atkins-friendly foods won't address all your needs.

- Keep some Atkins shakes and bars for a convenient, on-the-go breakfast or snack.
- Check out possibilities online, where most eateries post their menus.
- Find a sandwich bar or deli where you can pick up scrambled eggs or another suitable breakfast.
- Check out the nearest salad bar for good lunch choices.
- Research takeaway places or restaurants that deliver for dinner.

With your away-from-home meal sources identified and the right items in your kitchen, you'll be good to go. (For more on eating outside the home, see Chapter 10, "Dine Out with Ease".)

STOP CERTAIN SYMPTOMS BEFORE THEY START

A few small changes in your routine can help you avoid some unpleasant (and absolutely unnecessary) symptoms that could occur in the first couple of weeks as your body converts to a fat-burning machine. That's when some people experience fatigue, weakness, constipation, headaches, or leg cramps. Or light-headedness can occur when rising too quickly from a seated position, stepping out of a hot shower or hot bath, or simply engaging in household chores on a hot summer day. Some people complain that they feel "brain fog". Others refer to it as "Atkins flu".

These symptoms have nothing to do with eating fewer carbs or more protein and fat. Instead, they are the result of a deficit of sodium (salt). Eating the low-carb way is naturally diuretic. That's why you quickly lose those water pounds that can make you look bloated and puffy. Along with water, sodium and other minerals called electrolytes are flushed from your body. Just as an athlete needs to rehydrate and replace lost electrolytes when perspiring profusely, it's essential that you drink plenty of liquids and consume adequate salt to replace the water and sodium you're losing.

One of the reasons I emphasise eating a minimum amount of foundation vegetables each day is that they're full of both water and minerals, including sodium. They are also rich in fibre, which helps avoid constipation. But they may not contain enough sodium for you, especially if you've been eating a lot of salty snack foods until now or are fairly active. To ensure that you escape the above symptoms (or, at the very least, moderate them), I strongly suggest that you add a little extra sodium to your diet. (See "Sensitive to Salt?", below, if you have high blood pressure.) There are three ways you can do this. Each day, in addition to salting your food as you always have, add one of the following:

- An additional ½ teaspoon salt
- 2 tablespoons regular (not low-sodium) tamari (soya sauce)
- 480 ml (1 pint) regular (not low-sodium) beef, chicken, or vegetable stock – you can used the tinned kind or a stock cube in boiling water

---

SENSITIVE TO SALT?

If you have high blood pressure and take diuretics to control your blood pressure, talk to your GP before adding additional sodium to your diet. Many people find that their blood pressure drops naturally when they start eating the low-carb way, so monitor your blood pressure when you start Atkins and discuss any change in dosage with your GP.

If you're experiencing any of the symptoms described above, you can add another 5 grams of Net Carbs in the form of nuts or seeds or a small tin of tomato juice until you feel like yourself again. Then drop back to 20 grams of Net Carbs (and omit the nuts or tomato juice) to fast-track weight loss.

THE SCOOP ON SUGAR: MULTIPLE ALIASES

Like some criminals, sugar commits its offences under many names. Regardless of the name, sugar in foods and beverages quickly turns to blood sugar (and then fat) in your body. Some names indicate the source of the sugar: cane, date, grape, maple, or beet sugar. Others indicate colour: white, brown, yellow, or golden sugar. Some refer to texture: icing, caster, or granulated sugar. Other names imply minimal processing: raw, demerara, or muscovado. Some are familiar: caramel, honey, maple syrup, or molasses. Bottom line: they're all sugar. Also be on the lookout for these aliases on the labels of packaged foods:

- Agave syrup or crystals
- Barley malt
- Cane juice crystals
- Corn syrup, corn syrup solids, high-fructose corn syrup
- Dextran or dextrose
- Diastase, diastatic malt
- Fructose
- Fruit juice, fruit juice concentrate
- Galactose
- Glucose, glucose solids
- Golden syrup
- Lactose
- Maltose, maltol
- Refiner's syrup
- Rice syrup
- Sorghum syrup
- Sucrose
- Treacle

FREQUENTLY ASKED QUESTIONS

Q. Do I have to start Atkins in Phase 1?
A. No. You can start in any of the first three phases. If you have just a few pounds to lose, up to about 7 kg (15 lb), you can probably start in Phase 2 (Balancing) at 25 to 30 grams of Net Carbs a day. If you are heavier, you can also start here, but it could take considerably longer to lose weight without the kick start that you get in Phase 1. You can also begin in Phase 3 (Fine-Tuning) at, say, 45 grams of Net Carbs a day if you have very little weight to lose or are willing to shed it very slowly.

Q. Do I have to count carbs if I follow the meal plans exactly?
A. No. However, it's unlikely that you'll follow them to the letter day in and day out unless you eat every meal at home, so it's a good idea to use the Atkins Carb Counter. Also, if you aren't precise about serving size, you may be consuming more carbs than the meal plan

indicates. In any case, it's important to know how to count carbs as you start to add back more foods. Counting provides a double check that improves your likelihood of success from the start.

Q. Must I have two snacks a day?
A. Not necessarily. If you're having four or five small meals a day, you may not feel the need for snacks, but be very careful not to go more than four to six hours between meals. Instead, have a hot drink, perhaps a cup of broth.

Q. What is water weight loss?
A. The first few pounds you lose on any weight-loss programme are primarily water, and Atkins has a particularly diuretic effect. That's why it's essential to drink plenty of water and other fluids, eat your foundation vegetables, and take a multivitamin-mineral supplement to replace the electrolytes you'll be flushing out of your body along with the excess fluid. After the first few days you'll be losing primarily body fat.

Q. Can I eat as much protein and fat as I wish?
A. No. Eating excessive protein will make you sluggish and interfere with weight loss. Overeat fat and you'll burn it and not body fat for energy.

Q. Why do I have to drink so much water?
A. Most people are borderline dehydrated all the time. Drinking enough fluid helps flush toxins from your body, combats constipation and bad breath, lubricates your joints, and is important to your overall health. Staying hydrated also assists with weight loss. Remember, some of your water requirement can be satisfied with coffee, tea, or other clear beverages, including broth.

Q. Most bacon is sugar- or maple-cured. Does that mean I can't eat bacon?
A. Bacon is fine in moderation. Any residual sugar from the curing process in bacon, ham, or other pork products is burned off when you cook it.

Q. Why do the carb counts for some vegetables differ depending upon whether they're raw or cooked?
A. Cooking compacts vegetables such as spinach or cabbage significantly. Carb counts reflect the cooked amount. Chopping or grating a vegetable also compacts it more than slicing does, and that impacts the carb count as well.

Q. Can I have pudding in Phase 1?
A. Yes, as long as you get your quota of foundation vegetables and don't exceed your Net Carb daily limit. A pudding should contain no more than 3 grams of Net Carbs per serving. An Atkins Advantage bar or one of our pudding recipes is a good choice.

TIME TO EVALUATE YOUR PROGRESS

After seven days in Phase 1 (Kick-Start), weigh and measure yourself. If you've lost several kilos and centimetres, you've almost certainly lost fat in addition to the initial fluid loss. If you've lost only centimetres or more centimetres than kilos, don't worry. Centimetres often show up first and the kilos are sure to follow. Keep doing what you're doing! What if you lost just a kilo or two? That's still nothing to sneeze at. Check your measurements too. You may have made more progress there. And try to see the glass as half full. After all, you weigh less than you did a week ago. Also think about how your clothes are fitting. If you're disappointed with your rate of loss, ask yourself whether your expectations were reasonable. While some people can lose up to 7 kg (15 lb) in two weeks, weight-loss patterns differ significantly from one person to another. And even if you could banish a half kilo a day when you were in your twenties, it's unlikely you can do so in your forties. On the other hand, the heavier you are, the more quickly you'll lose weight. Men usually lose faster than women, as do physically active people. Hormonal issues can make weight loss difficult. If you're sure that you were doing everything by the book your first week on Atkins, take this dietary reality test:

1. *Are you counting grams of Carbs?* If you're just estimating or you're not taking serving size into consideration, there's a good chance you're overdoing the carbs and haven't kick-started

your fat-burning engine. Use your Atkins Carb Counter and track in your journal everything you eat.

2. *Are you skipping meals or going too long without eating?* If so, you may get ravenous and overeat. Be sure to eat a meal or snack every three or four hours.

3. *Did you consume less than 18 or more than 22 grams of Net Carbs each day?* Having too few or too many carbs can interfere with jump-starting fat burning.

4. *Are you drinking eight glasses of acceptable liquids?* If not, increase your intake, using such tricks as setting the alarm on your mobile phone or filling a litre container with water twice a day. Being dehydrated can slow fat burning and produce other unpleasant side effects.

5. *Did you eat a minimum of 12–15 grams of Net Carbs from the foundation vegetables list each day?* This is not negotiable for the reasons stated earlier. If you haven't been doing this, get with the programme and you'll see the weight start to melt away.

6. *Are you eating more than the recommended amount of protein?* Unless you're a very tall man, if you're eating more than 175 g (6 oz) of protein at a single meal, you're overdoing it. Review and follow the guidelines provided earlier in this chapter and weight loss should speed up.

7. *Are you holding back on fat?* Again, eating natural fats is essential to turn your body fat into your primary fuel source. Lose your fear of fat and lose your fat!

8. *Did you have more than three sweeteners a day?* Some people are more sensitive than others to sugar substitutes. Even the small amount of carbs in these products can interfere with weight loss in Phase 1. Cut down on sweeteners or omit them altogether for a week or two.

9. *Did you check the ingredients list of any packaged foods or condiments you ate?* If not, you may have unwittingly consumed some hidden sugars. Develop an eagle eye for reading labels!

10. *Are you taking any medications that could interfere with weight loss?* If so, review Chapter 2 and discuss with your GP.

If this checklist unearthed some misunderstandings about how to follow the programme that are impeding your progress, simply make the recommendedchangesasyouenterWeek2.Ifyouhaven'talreadydoneso, I can't overstate how important it is to keep a daily journal of what you eat. Doing so will allow you to quickly spot the problems cited above. Even small changes, such as using less sweeteners, can have a significant impact.

• • •

Now meet Mike D., who lost more than half his start weight and has kept it off for a decade. Then learn more about Phase 1 (Kick-Start) in Chapter 4. For starters, we'll look at ways to add variety to meals (especially breakfast), coordinate Atkins meals with family meals, and deal with some of the day to-day challenges of getting meals on the table and in your tummy.

HALF THE MAN HE WAS, AND BETTER FOR IT

VITAL STATS

Daily Net Carb intake:
   20–30 grams

Age: 62

Height: 160 cm (5 ft 3 in)

Before weight: 135 kg
   (21 st 4 lb)

After weight: 55 kg (8 st 9 lb)

Weight lost: 80 kg (177 lb)

In 2004 when audiovisual consultant Mike D. of Napa, California, told his GP he wanted gastric bypass surgery, he was informed that he first needed to lose 10 per cent of his 135 kg (21 st 4 lb). After two months on Atkins and minus 14 kg (30 lb), Mike decided to see if he could lose more weight without going under the knife. It took him

14 months to achieve that goal, and he's maintained his trim 55 kg (8 st 9 lb) transformation since then. Mike tells his story.

My wife and I renewed our marriage vows in Las Vegas in 2003 in front of an Elvis Presley impersonator. Our first wedding was in a grotto in Hawaii, but that wasn't the only difference.

The second time I weighed more than twice what I did when we married 15 years earlier! Now, as our 25th anniversary approaches, I'm back to the weight I was as a groom.

I wasn't into most sweets, but I really liked high-carb food like crisps, dips, and pies. I used to make a cherry cheesecake to die for. My workplace was sociable and we'd have lots of potlucks and were all into desserts. I'd tried cutting back but nothing gave fast enough weight-loss results. When my health maintenance organisation started paying for gastric bypass surgery, I decided I wanted the weight off once and for all. I knew that with my smoking – I had a pack-and-a-half to two-pack habit – and being overweight, I was likely to die before my time.

I looked at several weight-loss programmes, decided on Atkins, and stayed on a modified form of Induction the whole 14 months it took me to lose the extra weight. One thing that helped me stay the course was that I'd reward myself with a new Hawaiian shirt for every 4.5 kg (10 lb) I lost. When I started doing Atkins I had a 152-cm (60-in) waist and was wearing extra large shirts. My waist is now half what it was and I now wear a small or medium.

My wife and I share the cooking. While I was losing I ate mostly meat and salads. The rest of the family would also have baked potatoes, pasta, breads, and the like.

They were totally supportive about my doing Atkins. Later my wife lost the 16 kg (35 lb) she wanted to lose on the programme. She and I find it easy to eat out. For example, we'll order prime ribs at our favourite diner but skip the corn bread and order extra vegetables instead.

Basically, I eat meats, cheese, salads, and cooked vegetables. I especially like chef's salads with ranch dressing. Nowadays, my treats are peanuts, sugar-free chocolate sweets, and Atkins bars. I've also found a great brand of low-carb bread called MiRico. It's the first bread I've had in ten years and occasionally I'll have it with no sugar-added jam. I do the food shopping and read labels carefully.

I'm aware of my carb intake but don't count carbs anymore. I realise now that the real key to weight loss is not the number of calories consumed in a day but the amount of carbs. At first I thought that I was "dieting" and that after I'd lost weight I'd go back to eating the things I used to eat. But I've come to understand that to keep weight off, it has to be a lifestyle change. My food preferences have actually changed a lot and I feel healthier.

When I went back to my doctor after losing the weight, he was amazed. All my health markers were excellent. When I told him that I did it on Atkins, he was delighted it had worked. His parting words were, "I probably won't see much of you from now on."

Losing weight on Atkins and being successful in keeping it off long term came in handy when it was time to give up my 30-year smoking habit. I wish I could say my decision was personal, but my workplace instituted a no-smoking policy. So it was give it up or go off premises every time I took a cigarette break. I was concerned that I might regain weight after I stopped smoking, but fortunately, I haven't. I seem to be a permanently slim guy!

MAKE IT EASY

My advice to anyone with more than 45 kg (100 lb) to lose is to stay on Phase 1 longer than two weeks. —MD

CHAPTER 4

YOUR SECOND WEEK ON ATKINS

You're now on your eighth day of eating the Atkins way and are probably off and running. Give yourself a pat on the back and flash a high five! You've almost certainly shed some of that padding around your middle – belly fat is the first to go on Atkins – meaning there's a little less of you to love. Your real weight loss should pick up now that you're losing only fat and not water weight. If you experienced fatigue for a few days as you transitioned to burning mostly fat, chances are that has vanished. Almost everyone reports a burst of energy by Week 2, and many people feel a sense of exhilaration. Perhaps most amazing of all, you're experiencing that marvellous sense of being in control of your appetite. Life is good! Stick with Atkins and it's only going to get better.

By now you know the guidelines for Phase 1 (Kick-Start) and have a good understanding of what's on the menu for the first week (and perhaps longer). In this chapter I'll show you how to branch out a bit with more options for breakfast, lunch, dinner, and snacks, including a complete meal plan for the week. We'll also delve deeper into the details of daily life in this phase, such as how to integrate Atkins into family meals, and address some challenges you may already be experiencing or anticipating. Time is at a premium for all of us, so I know you're looking for ways to eat nutritious low-carb meals and snacks with a minimum of effort. Resolving these and other important issues from the start will build your confidence in the programme and strengthen your commitment to stay the course.

SOLVING THE BREAKFAST DILEMMA

Breakfast on Atkins can be the most dramatic change from your usual eating pattern. No wonder. Just compare the typical low-carb and low-fat breakfasts below. The latter contains the equivalent of 18 teaspoons sugar (approximately 90 g), and that doesn't include a teaspoon or two of sugar in coffee or tea and jam or marmalade on the toast. On the other hand, the low-carb breakfast of two eggs cooked with 85 g (3 oz) chopped onion and 30 g (1 oz) Cheddar cheese in 1 teaspoon olive oil,

TYPICAL LOW-CARB BREAKFAST
Western Omelet

| 2 eggs | 1 tablespoon chopped onions & 3 tablespoons red bell pepper | 2 oz bacon | 1/2 cup shredded Cheddar cheese | 1.2 teaspoons sugar (5g Net Carbs) |

TYPICAL HIGH-CARB/LOW-FAT BREAKFAST
Yogurt, Cereal, Toast, & OJ

| 6 oz low-fat yogurt | 1/2 cup granola | A slice of whole wheat toast | 4 oz glass of OJ | 18 teaspoons sugar (76g Net Carbs) |

and 55 g (2 oz) bacon or sausage contains just 4.2 grams of Net Carbs – the equivalent of a single teaspoon of sugar. (For more breakfast carb bombs, see "Sweets for Breakfast" on page 70.)

There are a number of tasty and filling choices for breakfast in the first two weeks on Atkins. Let's start with the obvious. Egg lovers are in luck, as it's perfectly fine to have two or three eggs every day.

- Enjoy eggs poached, fried, scrambled, baked, hard-boiled, soft-boiled, or made into omelettes or frittatas.
- Serve eggs with sliced tomato, grated cheese, a pat of goat's cheese, bacon, sausage, or vegetables (reheated leftovers are fine) such as cooked spinach, asparagus, or broccoli.
- Jazz them up with sugar-free salsa or guacamole.
- Try Eggs Parmesan (page 213) or Breakfast Casserole (page 221).
- Check out the Atkins recipe database for dozens more delectable egg dishes.

Okay, you like eggs. And they're great on the weekend when you can chill out, but not on rushed weekday mornings. Or there's no handy deli or sandwich shop where you can pick up some scrambled eggs or an omelette – hold the toast – on your way to work. How about these ideas?

- Keep hard-boiled eggs in the fridge. Peel a couple in the morning, slice in half, and drizzle with hot sauce or top with a little mayo and salt and pepper. Or have one plus an Atkins shake or bar. No time to eat at home? What could be more portable than a hard-boiled egg neatly packaged in its shell?
- Make devilled eggs the night before, flavouring them with curry powder, pesto, chopped chives, or dill.
- Make a crustless quiche, dividing the mixture into six portions and bake in muffin tins. After they're cooled, freeze in individual portions and then reheat in the oven or microwave.

EGGLESS BREAKFAST OPTIONS

Even confirmed egg-lovers have days when they simply want something else. Or perhaps even on a good day an egg is the last thing you want to see on your plate in the morning. What to do?

- Grab a tasty and convenient Atkins Day Break bar or shake.
- Check out the Atkins recipe database for Bacon, Tomato & Cheddar Stacks, Cheesy Breakfast Meatballs, Coffee Frappe and other tempting egg-free breakfast options.
- Breakfast sausages (or turkey or soya-based versions) make a hearty breakfast that cooks quickly. Stuff into portobello mushroom caps and grill. Or grill the sausage, stack with slices of mozzarella and tomato, and run under the grill again.
- Pan-fried back bacon also makes great breakfast stacks. How about one made with Cheddar cheese and salsa on the side?

THE SCOOP ON SUGAR: SWEETS FOR BREAKFAST

The typical breakfast is made with white flour and sugar. In cereals the sugar may be in the form of dehydrated berries, marshmallows, honey, or maple syrup, adding to the already high carb count of grains. Hot cereals are right up there as well, particularly packaged ones. Orange juice might as well be liquid sugar, and bananas are among the fruits highest in carbs. Bagels are outta sight!

Take a look at the carb minefield represented by a few breakfast faves:

SERVING	ITEM	GRAMS OF CARBS
1 packet	Instant cinnamon porridge	33
30 g serving *	Crunchy Nut Cornflakes	31
30 g serving *	Honey Nut Cheerios	29
45 g	Grape-Nuts	32
40 g *	Alpen	38
45 g *	Crunchy Nut Oat Granola	34
40 g *	Frosted Wheats	35
125 ml (4 fl oz)	Orange juice	12
240 ml (8 fl oz)	Skimmed milk	10
1 medium	Plain bagel	54
1	Strawberry Frosted Pop-Tart	35
2	Tesco Finest Waffles	25.4
2 slices	White bread	24
1 small	Banana	20

*With 125 ml semi-skimmed milk

- Pan-fry a flank, minute, or other small steak and serve with vegetable leftovers.
- Roll up sliced ham or another meat and/or cheese and a few other ingredients for a quick, satisfying, and portable breakfast. (See "Design a Roll-Up" on page 73, for more options.)
- Whip up a breakfast smoothie in no time in a blender, using sugar-free protein powder and unsweetened, unflavoured almond milk, soya milk, or coconut milk beverage. Add sugar-free cocoa powder or syrup and/or instant coffee granules. You can even hide some raw spinach or another leafy green in the mix. Pop in some ice cubes for a great frothy texture.
- Enjoy waffles and pancakes made with soya flour, flax meal, or coconut flour. Okay, pancakes and waffles are made with eggs, but I've never heard anyone turn them down for that reason! Check out Courgette–Pumpkin Spice Pancakes (page 217) and Chocolate Waffles (page 219). You can make waffles or pancakes on the weekend, freeze, and then defrost in a toaster oven or under the grill for speedy weekday breakfasts.

Frozen fully cooked pork or turkey bacon or sausages save time and minimise clean-up since most of the fat has been removed. Bacon comes in streaky and back rashers, and back medallions, or bits; sausage can be found as crumbles, patties, and links. Some frozen omelettes are also available, but do check the ingredients list and Nutrition Information panel to ensure they contain no added sugars or other unacceptable ingredients. Avoid bacon and sausage products cured with nitrates.

MAKE BREAKFAST AHEAD OF TIME

Many of the breakfast recipes on atkins.com and several of those in this book are ideal candidates for making in quantity and freezing in individual portions. For best results, keep the following in mind:

- If you're baking in muffin tins instead of a tart tin, reduce the oven temp by 10°C (25°F) or so and the cooking time by 15 minutes and check for doneness at that point.
- Let quiches, muffins, and other baked goods come to room temperature before wrapping in cling film and then aluminium foil

or a freezer bag, and freezing for up to three months. Label and date each package.

- Remove the item the night before and let it defrost in the fridge to reduce reheating time the next morning in a microwave or toaster oven.

LUNCH AND DINNER ON THE DOUBLE

The midday meal isn't the major hurdle that breakfast can be for most Atkins beginners. To reduce the carbs in most traditional lunch choices:

- Instead of, say, a turkey sandwich, ditch the bread and order a big salad topped with sliced turkey.
- Or have several roll-ups – they're as portable as a sandwich – using sandwich components minus the bread (see "Design a Roll-Up" on page 73). Your turkey sandwich could morph into a roll-up of slices of turkey filled with cheese, shredded lettuce, and sliced tomato. Yum!
- Deconstruct a cheeseburger or beef burger (get rid of the bun) and accompany it with a side salad. Some burger places now offer burgers wrapped in lettuce leaves.
- Any main-dish salad with 115–175 g (4–6 oz) of protein in the form of meat, poultry, fish, or shellfish makes a great lunch that can be prepared in minutes. If you put one together at a salad bar, be sure to pass on the noodles, raisins, sweetcorn relish, and other high-carb offerings. Our recipe developer has come up with five salad zingers, starting on page 236, suitable for all phases of Atkins. Also check atkins.com for more main-dish salads.

If a salad leaves you wanting a little something more, a cup of hot stock may do the trick, as would any soup made with foundation vegetables and/or protein, but minus noodles, rice, potatoes or other starchy veggies. A smaller salad and a light soup such as Cream of Romanesco Broccoli Soup (page 244) make a great combo too. A hearty soup, chowder, or stew such as No-Bean Chicken Chilli (page 245), Taco Soup (page 246), or Salmon Mushroom Chowder (page 249) makes a complete lunch. There are plenty more delicious main-dish soups in the Atkins recipe database.

When ordering soup in a restaurant, ask about the ingredients. Many places use flour or cornflour as a thickener and often sugar for flavour. Likewise, check the ingredients list in tinned or packaged soups. The Atkins Carb Counter lists a few acceptable choices. Dinner is actually the easiest meal to deal with as you move away from the standard Western diet full of carbs. When cooking from scratch, simply replace the potato, pasta, or rice you used to have with a second vegetable serving or salad alongside your protein choice. You'll find lots more ways to make meals easier in Part III, "It's All About Food".

DESIGN A ROLL-UP

Mix and match the ingredients below to put together your own combinations. Feel free to combine cheese and meat as wraps. (You can also double-wrap in a lettuce leaf.) Three or four roll-ups make a great no-cook breakfast or lunch. One would serve as a super snack.

WRAPS	SPREADS	CENTRES
Sliced ham	Aioli	Asparagus
Sliced roast beef	Mayonnaise	Cucumber
Sliced turkey breast	Mustard	Avocado
Sliced smoked salmon	Cream cheese	Jicama or water chestnuts
Emmental cheese	Soft goat's cheese	Daikon or radish
Provolone		Roasted red pepper
Egg mayonnaise		
Pickle slices or gherkin		
Prosciutto		

PHASE 1 SNACKS PDQ

In addition to an Atkins Advantage shake or bar bar-coded for Phase 1, the five snacks in the recipe section, and the old Atkins standbys of olives, half a Hass avocado, jerky (cured without sugar or nitrates), and pork rinds, here are some easy and satisfying alternatives. None contains more than 3 grams of Net Carbs per serving.

- A serving of red pepper or courgette slices, cherry tomatoes, radishes, or almost any raw foundation vegetable with 1 tablespoon ranch, blue cheese, Italian, or other low-carb dressing
- 30 g (1 oz) of string cheese
- Celery stick stuffed with salmon cream cheese
- Cucumber "boat" filled with tuna mayonnaise
- A lettuce leaf wrapped round grated Cheddar cheese
- Prawn cocktail with full-fat mayonnaise and a dash of hot sauce
- Two slices of tomato topped with chopped fresh basil and grated mozzarella and run under the grill for a minute

WEEK-AT-A-GLANCE WEEK 2 MEAL PLAN

On pages 76–7 you'll find another week's worth of delicious, easy-to-prepare meals suitable for Phase 1. You'll continue to follow the first rung on the Carb Ladder (page 14), eating protein, foundation vegetables, and acceptable Phase 1 dairy products. Review the suggestions in this chapter for modifying the Week 1 meal plan with recipes in this book and the online database. Or substitute any meal suggestion from the earlier meal plan. The shopping list for this week's plan (below) includes only six new items, which appear in boldface italics. You'll also need to replenish your supplies of fresh foods and perhaps some other items. Be sure to adjust your shopping list if you've modified the meal plan.

TIME TO EVALUATE YOUR PROGRESS

After two weeks on Atkins, you're practically an old hand! By now you're probably reaching your stride, losing centimetres and kilos. I'll bet you can now zip up your jeans all the way again! Once more, take your measurements and weigh yourself. Why are your measurements so important? Assuming that you're exercising, you may be gaining lean body mass and losing fat. Because muscle is denser than fat, the scale can be deceiving. How your clothes fit is another useful calculation. Even if your weight remains stable for a week or so, if your jeans zip up more easily, you're losing fat.

If all went well during your first week, in all likelihood you continued to lose weight this week. If so, you're definitely burning fat for

SHOPPING LIST FOR WEEK 2

WEEK 2

PROTEINS	DAIRY/CHEESE	VEGETABLES	SAUCES/ PRODUCTS CONDIMENTS	ATKINS
Steak or Beef Burgers	Butter	Hass Avocados	Blue Cheese Dressing*	Atkins Bars
Chicken	Cheddar Cheese	Green Beans	Salsa*	Atkins Shakes
Eggs	Mozzarella	Cauliflower	Creamy Italian Dressing*	Atkins fusilli and penne
Ham or Pork Chops	Black Pepper Cheddar Cheese	Celery	Mayonnaise or Tartare Sauce*	
Tinned Tuna or Fish Fillet		Red Pepper	Ranch Dressing*	
Bacon or Sausages			Lettuce/Salad Leaves	Vinaigrette*
		Tomatoes	Extra-Virgin Olive Oil	

* Select sauces and condiments with no added sugar.

energy. You've probably also banished cravings for unsuitable foods, are in control of your appetite, feel energised, and have said good bye to any annoying symptoms if you ever had them. Keep up the good work. If you uncovered some glitches after the first week and have corrected them, the chances are good that your results have improved. It may have taken you a little longer to spark your fat-burning metabolism, but now you're on your way.

But what if you have made all of the recommended changes that could have been hindering weight loss in the first week but the weight refuses to budge? Sad to say, some people are highly resistant to weight loss, and you may simply be a slow starter. In addition to the issues discussed earlier, here are some possible reasons and suggestions for overcoming them:

- You're simply eating too much despite thinking your portions are appropriately sized. Review the guidelines on page 48 one more time and, rather than estimate, actually measure your portions and record them.

Atkins Phase 1 (Kick-Start) Meal Plan at 20 g NC/day: Week 2

	MONDAY	TUESDAY	WEDNESDAY	THURSDAY

BREAKFAST	2 eggs
	90 g chopped pepper
	30 g mozzarella cheese
	120 g bacon or sausage
	
	Net Carbs: 2.9 g; FV: 2.2 g
		Atkins Advantage Café
		    Royal RTD & Atkins Day
		    Break Chocolate Chip
		    Crisp Bar
		
		Net Carbs: 3.4 g; FV: 0 g
			2 eggs
			45 g chopped pepper
			½ avocado
			30 g Cheddar cheese
			2 tbsp salsa
			Net Carbs: 5.7 g; FV: 4 g
				60 g bacon or sausage
				90 g chopped pepper
				75 g chopped onion
				30 g Cheddar cheese
				
				Net Carbs: 5.6 g; FV: 5.3 g

SNACK	Atkins Vanilla Shake Mix
	
	Net Carbs: 2.8 g; FV: 0 g
		90 g sliced pepper
		2 tbsp Blue Cheese
		    Dressing*
		Net Carbs: 3.4 g; FV: 2.7 g
			1 small tomato
			60 g mozzarella cheese
			
			Net Carbs: 2.5 g; FV: 2.5 g
				Atkins Day Break Strawberry
				    Yoghurt RTD
				
				Net Carbs: 3 g; FV: 0 g

LUNCH	115–175 g chicken
	1 small tomato
	55 g mixed lettuce
	2 tbsp Blue Cheese
	    Dressing*
	
	Net Carbs: 4.6 g; FV: 3.8 g
		115–175 g steak or
		    beefburger
		100 g mixed lettuce
		2 tbsp Ranch Dressing*
		
		Net Carbs: 3.4 g; FV: 2.7 g
			Atkins Advantage Chocolate
			    and Orange Bar
			
			Net Carbs: 1.9 g; FV: 0 g
				115–175 g chicken
				55 g mixed greens
				45 g sliced pepper
				2 tbsp Vinaigrette*
				
				Net Carbs: 2.7 g; FV: 2.2 g

SNACK	1 medium tomato 60 g Cheddar cheese Net Carbs: 5.3 g; FV: 3.3 g	Atkins Advantage Dark Chocolate Crunch Bar Net Carbs: 3.7 g; FV: 0 g	45 g sliced pepper 2 tbsp Ranch Dressing* Net Carbs: 2.6 g; FV: 1.9 g	1 small tomato 30 g Cheddar cheese Net Carbs: 3.5 g; FV: 2.5 g

DINNER	115–175 g steak or
	    beefburger
	100 g cauliflower florets
	1 tbsp butter
	55 g mixed lettuce
	1 celery stick
	2 tbsp Vinaigrette*
	
	Net Carbs: 5.9 g; FV: 5.5 g
		115–175 g tinned tuna or
		    fish fillet
		55 g mixed lettuce
		½ avocado
		45 g mozzarella cheese
		2 tbsp Creamy Italian
		    Dressing*
		55 g green beans
		1 tbsp butter
		Net Carbs: 7.1 g; FV: 6.8 g
			115–175 g chicken
			55 g green beans
			1 tbsp butter
			100 g mixed lettuce
			½ avocado
			2 tbsp Creamy Italian
			    Dressing*
			
			Net Carbs: 6.3 g; FV: 6.1 g
				115–175 g ham or pork
				    chop
				100 g cauliflower florets
				30 g Cheddar cheese
				100 g mixed lettuce
				2 tbsp Ranch Dressing*
				
				Net Carbs: 7 g; FV: 5.9 g

	Total Net Carbs: 21.5 g
	Total Net Carbs from FV:
	    14.8 g
		Total Net Carbs: 21 g
		Total Net Carbs from FV:
		    12.2 g
			Total Net Carbs: 19 g
			Total Net Carbs from FV:
			    14.5 g
				Total Net Carbs: 21.8 g
				Total Net Carbs from FV:
				    15.9 g

FRIDAY	SATURDAY	SUNDAY
2 eggs ½ avocado 30 g Cheddar cheese 2 tbsp salsa	2 small tomatoes 60 g bacon or sausage 30 g Cheddar cheese	Atkins Day Break Strawberry Crisp Bar
Net Carbs: 4.6 g; FV: 2.9 g	Net Carbs: 5.3 g; FV: 4.9 g	Net Carbs: 3 g; FV: 0 g
Atkins Day Break Cappuccino Nut Bar	45 g sliced pepper 2 tbsp Ranch Dressing*	2 celery sticks 60 g Cheddar cheese
Net Carbs: 3.5 g; FV: 0 g	Net Carbs: 2.6 g; FV: 1.9 g	Net Carbs: 2.7 g; FV: 2 g
115–175 g tinned tuna or fish fillet 2 tbsp mayonnaise or tartar sauce 1½ celery sticks 150 g mixed lettuce ½ avocado 2 tbsp Creamy Italian Dressing*	Atkins Advantage Peanut Caramel Bar	115–175 g steak or beefburger 55 g mixed lettuce 1 small tomato 45 g sliced pepper ½ avocado 2 tbsp Ranch Dressing*
Net Carbs: 7 g; FV: 6.9 g	Net Carbs: 2.8 g; FV: 0 g	Net Carbs: 7.1 g; FV: 6.5 g
Atkins Advantage Milk Chocolate RTD	1 small tomato 60 g mozzarella cheese	Atkins Chocolate Shake Mix
Net Carbs: 1.3 g; FV 0 g	Net Carbs: 2.5 g; FV: 2.5 g	Net Carbs: 3 g; FV: 0 g
115–175 g chicken 55 g mixed lettuce ½ small tomato 2 tbsp Vinaigrette*	115–175 g steak or beefburger 55 g green beans 1 tbsp olive oil 55 g mixed lettuce ½ avocado 2 tbsp Blue Cheese Dressing*	115–175 g chicken 100 g cauliflower florets 1 tbsp butter 55 g mixed lettuce 2 tbsp Creamy Italian Dressing*
Net Carbs: 3 g; FV: 2.5 g	Net Carbs: 5.4 g; FV: 4.7 g	Net Carbs: 4.8 g; FV: 4.5 g
Total Net Carbs: 19.4 g Total Net Carbs from FV: 12.3 g	Total Net Carbs: 18.6 g Total Net Carbs from FV: 14 g	Total Net Carbs: 20.6 g Total Net Carbs from FV: 13 g

- You have high insulin levels. Insulin is the fat-storing hormone. It may simply take you longer to initiate fat burning by controlling carb intake.
- You have an underactive thyroid. If this has been a problem in the past or you suspect it may be now, discuss it with your GP.
- Your menstrual period is interfering with weight loss. Some women lose very slowly or not at all right before their period.
- Certain medications may interfere with weight loss. Review the list on page 38 and discuss alternatives with your GP.
- You're sedentary. Begin some form of exercise, such as walking or swimming, to see if that gets the pounds moving along with you.

TEAM UP

Whether it's improving your tennis game or slimming down, it's definitely easier to achieve any goal if you're working with someone who has your back. That's what friends are for. You'll be able to celebrate each other's victories as well as help each other regain equilibrium when forward momentum is lacking. A friend also helps keep you in line, perhaps talking you off the ledge when a jam doughnut beckons after a stressful day. In an ideal world, your friend would be your gender and age, have about the same amount of weight to lose, and live down the street. That said, if you're both doing Atkins, your significant other might be a great partner. A friend or relative in another town could do too, as could someone you meet in an Atkins chat room. With Skype, email, instant messaging, or tweets, you may never meet face-to-face with the person who's sharing your journey.

If you're having trouble sticking with the programme, an Atkins friend can be a huge help. If your problem is more one of perception than of compliance, accept that although you're losing more slowly than you'd hoped, you're heading in the right direction. For more on troubleshooting in Phase 1 (Kick-Start), see the FAQs that follow.

FREQUENTLY ASKED QUESTIONS

Q. Can I eat more carbs one day if I cut back the next?
A. By maintaining a constant level of carb intake from day to day, you're more likely to keep your blood sugar on an even keel. But a range of 3 or 4 grams of Net Carbs from one day to the next should not create a problem as long as your average intake is consistent. If you do over-indulge one day, simply return to your current level the next day.

Q. Why can't I do Atkins during the week and then take the weekend off?
A. Doing so will mean that you're consistently returning to a primarily blood-sugar metabolism for two days. It then takes several days to reignite your fat-burning engine. Stopping and starting, known as "carb cycling", will lessen the likelihood that you'll lose weight or keep it off.

Q. Will drinking caffeinated beverages interfere with weight loss?
A. Caffeine itself doesn't slow weight loss. Drinking a few cups of coffee or tea each day actually produces numerous health benefits. However, have your beverages without sugar or honey. Non-caloric sweeteners are okay, but have no more than three a day. Also lighten these beverages with double cream, single cream or acceptable dairy substitutes, not milk.

Q. Can I consume beer, wine, or other alcohol in Phase 1?
A. No. However, once you transition to Phase 2, you can consume moderate amounts of most alcoholic beverages, assuming it doesn't interfere with weight loss, as we'll discuss in Chapter 5.

Q. If the objective is to stay at 20 grams of Net Carbs a day, why can't I have Atkins bars and shakes or a slice of bread instead of all those vegetables?
A. You're not just tracking your carb intake; you're also aiming for a well-balanced meal plan full of vitamins and other nutrients provided by vegetables, along with fibre to help manage your hunger. One slice of bread might represent the balance of your daily carb intake in Phase 1, which would put your blood sugar back on the roller coaster.

Q. Why can't I drink tomato or orange juice with my breakfast?
A. The juicing process removes all or most of the fibre in fruit and vegetables, concentrating the sugar hit. You'll be able to introduce tomato juice in Phase 2. In Phase 3, oranges and other citrus fruits are acceptable.

Q. Why is cream allowed in Phase 1 but not milk?
A. Strange as it may seem, milk is higher in carbs than cream, thanks to the lactose (a form of sugar). In Phase 2 you can reintroduce small amounts of whole milk. Or dilute cream with some water, if you prefer.

Q. I'm experiencing cravings for sweets and other high-carb foods such as muffins, bread, and crisps. How do I stay in control of my appetite?
A. Most likely your blood-sugar levels have not yet stabilised, which usually occurs after the fifth day on Atkins. Once you're burning fat for energy, it acts as a natural appetite suppressant. Sometimes women have cravings right before their menstrual period. Or you may be going too long between meals or snacks, eating foods that contain hidden sugars or grains, or not consuming enough fat. When you experience cravings for high-carb foods, have an Atkins bar or shake, half a Hass avocado, some cheese, or some olives instead. Hunger and cravings can also be confused with thirst, so drink up.

In the next chapter, we'll tackle the all-important question of the right time to move on to Phase 2 (Balancing) of the New Atkins Diet. For some of you it's likely to be after two weeks on the programme. Or you may prefer to wait several weeks or even several months. It's your decision and many factors come into play, but I'll give you the pros and cons for each path so you can make the decision that's right for you.

Meanwhile, turn the page to meet Patricia O., who found some weight returning after she'd kept it off for years. When she came to understand the changes she needed to make in order to stay on top of her weight and returned to her exercise regime, the excess weight beat a hasty retreat.

ATKINS PLUS EXERCISE ADDS UP
TO SUCCESS

VITAL STATS

Daily Net Carb intake:
25 grams
Age: 25
Height: 165 cm (5 ft 5 in)

Before weight: 114 kg (18 st)
After weight: 67 kg
(10 st 8 lb)
Lost: (47 kg) 101 pounds

Nurse and aspiring physician Patricia O. lost weight six years ago on Atkins and kept it off while she was in nursing school. But after graduation she returned home to Houston, where juggling a demanding job while taking the college courses necessary to apply to medical school made it hard to stay on track. Finding time to exercise was almost impossible. It's not surprising that some of the lost weight returned. Working with the support of an Atkins nutritionist online, Patricia was able to banish the weight again and begin a maintenance programme she could stick to despite her hectic schedule. Here's her story.

I've dealt with weight issues all my life. I remember once being teased so badly at school for being heavy that I came home crying. When I told my father what the other kids had said to me, instead of comforting me, he agreed with them. My father's attitude didn't help my self-image. Once he and I were shopping and in front of a group of other girls, he said, "How come you can't look like them? Just look at yourself." It wasn't until later on in my life that I realised that was his way to motivate me to change my eating habits. Of course, losing weight was solely dependent on me to decide that I'd had enough of feeling bad about myself. Meanwhile, my mother would tell me to eat. I felt pulled in two directions.

I've always been an emotional eater, and I loved sweets, potatoes, macaroni cheese, and anything white. By the time I graduated from high school, I weighed 91 kg (14 st 5 lb). Then, instead of the usual "fresher 7 kg (15 lb)", I gained 23 kg (50 lb) in my first year of nursing school, and my emotional state was terrible. Another nursing student introduced me to Atkins and told me what to eat and not to eat. Doing Atkins put me more in control, so I was able to lose the excess weight and keep it off for three and a half years. I also began working out at the same time I started Atkins. In the process, I overcame my insecurities.

One thing I knew for sure was that I never wanted to go back to that dark place where I was before!

That made it all the more upsetting when I started regaining lost weight. I was frustrated but knew I had to do something. I had completed nursing school and was working full-time. I had decided to apply to medical school – I want to go into cardiology – but needed to take postgrad courses in physics and organic chemistry. There didn't seem to be enough hours in the day to handle work, college, and homework, plus establish a routine that allowed me to eat properly and exercise. I was doing Atkins during the week but bingeing on carbs on the weekend. Not surprisingly, I couldn't lose the 5 kg (12 lb) I'd regained.

I now realise that I wasn't really doing Atkins – or I wasn't doing it correctly. I'd never read a book about why and how it works. And I didn't get it that Phase 1 was not the whole Atkins programme. I thought I would just have to eat that way for the rest of my life to keep the weight off. After reading *The New Atkins for a New You* and getting a pep talk from an Atkins nutritionist, I was motivated to get on the right track. I started keeping a journal, added nuts to my meals, and slowly added other carb foods. I'm back to running 8 km (5 miles) five times a week. I now know that staying active is key to maintaining my weight. Even 30 minutes a day makes a huge difference. My mood has lifted, and best of all, I've lost the weight I regained. And it wasn't even that hard! My next goal is to lose another 2.2 kg (5 lb). And now that I'm doing everything right, I know I will get there!

MAKE IT EASY

Always plan ahead. If you don't have the right food with you at all times, you may be tempted to eat whatever is handy. *–PO*

CHAPTER 5

WHAT'S NEXT? TRANSITION TO PHASE 2 – OR NOT

After two weeks on Atkins, it's decision time. Assuming you've been following the programme correctly and have lost weight over the last two weeks, you can choose to remain in Phase 1 (Kick-Start) or move to Phase 2 (Balancing). Although you should spend a minimum of two weeks in the first phase to train your body to burn fat, initiating weight loss, there's no maximum limit. In the second phase, you'll get into the steady rhythm of weight loss that will carry you until you're 7 kg (15 lb) from your goal weight. By then, you'll understand how your body reacts to certain foods and to gradual increases in carb intake. The decision about when you start to move up the Carb Ladder is a purely personal one. Many people come to regard Phase 1 as a "security blanket", because for the first time in years they feel in control of what they put in their mouth. And their continuing positive results reinforce this inaction. However, at some point weight loss is bound to slow, even if you stay at 20 grams of Net Carbs a day. It can be a false security to feel that you cannot leave this phase. In the long run, it's essential to find out what you can eat while maintaining a healthy weight. Moving up the Carb Ladder enables you to do this. Learning a way to eat for a lifetime is the real objective of Atkins.

FACTORS TO CONSIDER

That said, you may remain in Phase 1 as long as you want, assuming you don't become bored with the food choices or get within 7 kg

(15 lb) of your goal weight. In fact, there's no health risk associated with staying in this phase indefinitely. (See "Carb Balancing – Steps to Weight Loss" on page 15 to visualise the two paths, known as Fast Track and Slow and Steady, described below.) The trick is not to get stuck there. Feel free to hang out in Phase 1 longer than two weeks if you have a lot of weight to lose. Weight loss typically slows after the initial dramatic drop that occurs when you switch to burning primarily fat for energy. But that natural slowdown is actually a good thing, as we'll discuss here. In addition to reducing the possibility of boredom, there's another reason why staying too long in Phase 1 can be a problem: you'll have no place to go if and when – and it's almost inevitable – you experience a weight-loss plateau. That's because you can't drop below 20 grams of Net Carbs a day without sacrificing foundation vegetables, which is not negotiable. (We'll discuss plateauing in Chapter 6.)

THE FAST TRACK

If you're motivated by quick weight loss and thrive on structure and a minimum of choices, you may choose to stay in Phase 1 beyond two weeks. To make this process easier, as well as set the stage for when you do decide to move on:

- Continue to consume 20 grams of Net Carbs a day beyond the first two weeks.
- Try adding nuts and seeds to your list of acceptable foods. Nuts are full of protein and healthy fats and are relatively low in carbs, thanks to their high fibre content.
  - To make it easy, simply follow the meal plans on pages 54–5 and 74–5, swapping out 3 grams of Net Carbs from other foods, such as 85 g (3 oz) of green beans, a smallish tomato, or 115 g (4 oz) salad leaves, for 3 grams of Net Carbs of nuts or seeds, but without letting your intake of foundation vegetables dip below 12 grams of Net Carbs. (You'll still have 5 grams for Atkins bars and shakes, sweeteners, dressings, or condiments.)
  - As a quick guide, 3 grams of Net Carbs of nuts or seeds translates as: 30 almonds; 3 tablespoons macadamia nuts; 2 tablespoons peanut butter; 2 tablespoons shelled pistachios; or 4 tablespoons shelled sunflower seeds; 24 walnut halves come in at 3.4 grams.

  - Portion out nuts and seeds in advance to avoid overeating. A couple of tablespoons of walnuts, almonds, pecans, or pumpkin seeds make a great snack. Or top a salad with sunflower seeds or chopped walnuts. You can also now have other nut and seed butters (stuff them into celery sticks) or coconut, almond, and other nut flours (available in the baking section or speciality foods aisle of the supermarket).
- Move to Phase 2 (Balancing) no later than when you're within 7 kg (15 lb) of your goal weight. At that point it's time to start moving to a permanent way of eating by introducing foods higher up the Carb Ladder.

Fast Track pros: Speedier weight loss, greater structure, and fewer choices, meaning fewer opportunities for temptation.

Fast Track cons: Boredom; no options for moving past a plateau without reducing Net Carbs below the recommended level, which can be extremely frustrating and demotivating.

SLOW AND STEADY

Alternatively, you may choose to lose the bulk of your weight in Phase 2 (Balancing), which Dr Atkins dubbed Ongoing Weight Loss (OWL). If you're comfortable with a slower, steadier rate of weight loss, after two weeks (or a few more) start to climb the Carb Ladder (page 14). The gradual increase in Net Carb intake and reintroduction of new foods allows you to continue to shave off pounds and inches, maintain appetite control, and feel energetic. You'll also gradually come to understand which, if any, foods trigger cravings for more of the same and/or interfere with weight loss.

You may find that you're comfortable at a relatively low level of Net Carbs a day, perhaps 25 to 35 grams, which is not all that different from Kick-Start but does allow you to eat such delicious, nutritious food as nuts and seeds (see the meal plan for 25 grams of Net Carbs on pages 101–101, for easy ways to add them) and then berries, melon, and cherries (see the meal plan for 30 grams of Net Carbs on pages 112–113 for easy ways to add them). Next you'll move on to Greek yoghurt and fresh cheeses (see page 94 for easy ways to add these "new" foods). Or you may find you can go considerably higher, say 50 or 60 grams of Net Carbs or even more, which will allow you to include legumes and some vegetable juices.

The balancing process enables you to find what works for you. Understanding your carb tolerance is the bridge from a weight-loss diet to a diet for life. This process can involve some stops and starts as you increase the variety of foods, but it's essential to understanding your unique metabolism. After all, wouldn't you rather lose a little more slowly and keep the weight off for good than lose rapidly by staying in Phase 1, reach your goal weight, and then regain those lost kilos because you never learnt how to eat for the long run? Think of Atkins as a marathon rather than a sprint and you'll understand the rationale for losing the bulk of your weight in Phase 2 (Balancing).

Slow and Steady pros: More variety in what you can eat; more options for moving past a plateau because you can always return to a lower level of carb intake; easier shift to a sustainable way of eating.

Slow and Steady cons: Slightly slower weight loss; having more food choices may be too tempting or confusing.

WHICH PATH IS RIGHT FOR YOU?

Both these strategies will allow you to lose weight, but select the one that works best for you in the long run. By that I mean the option that will allow you to lose the weight – and then keep it off – while enjoying a satisfying way of eating. As you consider whether to leave the relative security of Induction to move on to Ongoing Weight Loss, ask yourself these questions.

- *Is routine important to you?* Are you in the habit of eating the same foods day after day? If your attitude is "Just tell me what to eat and I'm fine", you may actually find Atkins easier with a shorter list of acceptable foods, at least initially. Or do you get bored eating the same meals over and over again and delight in experimenting with new foods and new recipes?
- *Are you a tortoise or a hare?* Are you willing to take a bit longer to make the journey easier, or are you in a rush to get to your destination? Do you really miss eating berries or having a glass of

wine, or can you put up with those limitations for the time being to get your weight under control sooner?

- *Do you miss certain foods?* If you might have a hard time moderating your intake of some foods beyond the first rungs of the Carb Ladder, you may want to hold off for now. Or if there's nothing there you can't live without for the time being, you may decide to wait. Or perhaps being able to have yoghurt and berries for breakfast will make it easier to stay with Atkins.
- *What else is going on in your life?* If you're juggling work, a family, and study, for example, you may want to simplify things by staying with Phase 1 for the time being. Or perhaps for you, being able to eat a greater variety of foods is easier when other aspects of your life are stressful.

IT'S NOT JUST ABOUT WEIGHT

As you evaluate your experience in the first two weeks of Induction, look beyond just the changes in your weight and waistline. Those numbers are probably why you started Atkins, but consider other markers as well.

- If you have high blood pressure, has your blood pressure dropped? If your new way of eating is lowering it naturally and making you feel light-headed, be sure to talk to your GP – you likely need to reduce the dosage of your medication.
- If you are pre-diabetic or have Type 2 diabetes, have your blood-sugar levels improved? If so, it's crucial that you communicate that to your doctor in case it requires a change in your insulin or other medication dosage.
- Have your aches and pains diminished or vanished?
- Has your mood lifted?
- Are you in control of your appetite?

These factors are all part of the larger picture of how eliminating added sugar and other empty carbohydrates from your diet can improve your health and wellbeing. Even if your weight loss has been minimal, these indicators are clear evidence that Atkins is working for you.

TIME TO EXERCISE THE FITNESS OPTION?

Whether or not you decide to remain in Phase 1, after two weeks you may now want to add physical fitness to your weight-loss programme. Regular physical activity is important for numerous reasons, among them:

- Maintaining cardiovascular health
- Keeping bones strong
- Lowering high blood pressure
- Boosting your metabolism
- Improving sleep quality
- Helping coordination and balance as you get older.

If you already exercise regularly, whether walking briskly, taking Zumba or spinning classes, working out in a gym, or whatever, by all means continue to do so as long as your energy levels remain high. It's not a good idea to simultaneously increase your current activity level or begin an intense fitness programme as you start Atkins. However, once you get the burst of energy that usually occurs sometime within the first two weeks, ramp up your physical activity gradually.

What if you haven't been in the habit of exercising? I suggest you wait until you are comfortable with Atkins before starting or resuming a routine. After two weeks in Phase 1, that time may be right for you. If you've never been a "fitness freak" but want to test the waters, walking or swimming are the best ways to begin. Start small, perhaps a ½ -km (¼-mile) walk before dinner or a few laps in the pool, and then increase your distances gradually. If you're extremely heavy, swimming is an excellent choice, because it causes minimal impact on your joints. The same goes for exercises you can do sitting in a chair.

Does that mean you must start some form of exercise after two weeks on Atkins whether or not you remain in Phase 1 or advance to Phase 2? No way. If your energy levels are low or you simply aren't comfortable getting physical until you reduce your size, that's your choice. When and which kind of activity are personal decisions, but fitness is the natural partner to Atkins. So don't be surprised when I bring up exercise again in later chapters. Sooner or later you'll probably agree. As you'll hear from our success stories, most people found that as they slimmed down on Atkins, they became more interested in physical activity. Several of them, including Troy (page 123), have embraced competitive sports with a passion. Natalie (page 164) exercises "every single day, no matter what". Meanwhile, Joe (page 188), who has taught tae kwon do for years, no longer experiences excruciating pain after working out now that there is 91 kg (200 lb) less of him!

Physical activity helps some people lose weight, but not everyone. However, it will reliably help you maintain your weight loss over the long term. The combination of following Atkins while engaging in regular physical exercise benefits body and mind by:

- Increasing your energy levels
- Helping unlock your fat stores
- Inducing calmness
- Reducing stress
- Firming up flab
- Empowering you with a sense of mastery.

Weight training or other strength-building exercise also helps build muscle, giving your body a more defined appearance. As a result, your clothes fit better. And the less fat and more muscle you have, the higher your metabolism, which means you burn more fat even when you're sitting or sleeping.

MOVING TO PHASE 2

If you've made the decision to take the Slow and Steady Track by stepping up to Phase 2 (Balancing) sooner rather than later, you'll most likely spend the greatest amount of time in this phase as you continue to slim down. That's why it's designed to help you change habits as you gradually move towards a permanent way of eating. You'll experience greater freedom in this phase than in Phase 1 (Kick-Start). The trick is to exercise that freedom without undoing your initial results. The best way to handle that juggling act, what we call finding your personal carb balance, is to move slowly and deliberately up the Carb Ladder.

I can almost guarantee that if you rush to add back as many different foods as fast as you can, you'll stall your fat-burning engine. Worse, you could become discouraged and even give up on losing weight. Not to worry. I'm not going to let that happen to you. Nor do you have to retreat to the "safety net" of Phase 1. Here's how to succeed as you proceed up the Carb Ladder.

- Continue to consume a minimum of 12–15 daily grams of Net Carbs as foundation vegetables. Also continue to avoid foods with added sugar, have eight glasses of water or other acceptable fluids each day, and go no longer than three or four hours between meals or snacks, spreading out your carb intake across the day.
- Reintroduce food groups one by one, following the Carb Ladder. Depending on your metabolism and weight-loss goal, this may be at weekly intervals, every couple of weeks, or even longer.
- Add back carb foods within each rung of the ladder one by one as well. For example, reintroduce walnuts but gauge their impact, if any, before reintroducing almonds.
- Increase your overall daily Net Carb intake in 5-gram increments at weekly, biweekly, or even monthly intervals, whichever works best for you.
- Continue to track your daily Net Carb intake in your journal, also noting any new foods so that you can tell if they are stalling your progress.
- Continue to weigh and measure yourself weekly.

You may be reassured to see how similar Phase 1 (Kick-Start) is to Phase 2 (Balancing) initially. Again, proceeding slowly and deliberately will make it easy to move from one phase to the next. In the following chapter, we'll go into greater detail on what to expect as you move forwards, how to manage the food reintroduction process, and how to evaluate your responses to more carbs and a greater variety of foods.

CLIMBING THE CARB LADDER

In Phase 2, you'll start looking for your personal carb balance, increasing your Net Carb intake as you gradually reintroduce the foods on the five Phase 2 (Balancing) rungs of the Carb Ladder. (Since you can add nuts and seeds if you stay more than two weeks in Phase 1, they are not shown below.)

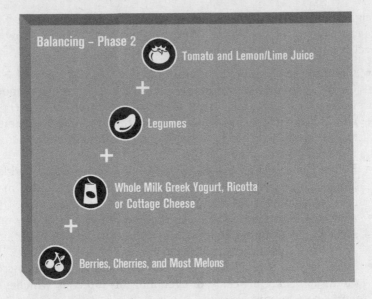

Balancing – Phase 2

Tomato and Lemon/Lime Juice

+

Legumes

+

Whole Milk Greek Yogurt, Ricotta or Cottage Cheese

+

Berries, Cherries, and Most Melons

ACCEPTABLE PHASE 2 FOODS

Now, let's take a closer look at the acceptable Phase 2 foods incorporated in the Balancing process. Understand that you may not be able to reintroduce all of them in this phase. Nor may you be interested in eating all of them. The following lists are representative of each rung on the Carb Ladder. For a more complete list of options, complete with serving sizes and Net Carb gram counts, see the printed, online, or mobile app Atkins Carb Counter.

NUTS AND SEEDS

Peanuts, cashews, and soy "nuts" are not true nuts, but they can also be reintroduced in Phase 2. Avoid chestnuts, which are very high in carbs, and salted nuts, which are notoriously difficult to eat in moderation. Also avoid products such as Nutella, which contains added sugars.

- Almonds
- Brazil nuts
- Cashews
- Coconut (fresh or grated and unsweetened)
- Macadamias
- Hazelnuts
- Peanuts
- Pecans
- Pine nuts
- Pistachios
- Pumpkin seeds
- Sesame seeds
- Soy "nuts"
- Sunflower seeds
- Walnuts

BERRIES, CHERRIES, AND MOST MELONS

The fruits suitable for OWL are lower in Net Carbs than most other fruits because their fibre content is relatively high and fruit sugar content is relatively low. Still, have small portions and always accompany them with fat or protein. The following fruits can be eaten fresh, frozen (as long as they're unsweetened), or tinned in water or juice (but not syrup). You can also have 1-tablespoon portions of berry or cherry preserves that have no added sugar and are sweetened only with acceptable sweeteners.

- Blackberries, blueberries, boysenberries, fresh currants, gooseberries, loganberries, raspberries, and strawberries
- Cherries, sour or sweet

- Unsweetened cranberries and cranberry sauce made with acceptable sweeteners only
- Melon: cantaloupe, galia, and honeydew (but not watermelon).

MAKE IT EASY

Always have berries or other Phase 2 fruits with cheese, cream, Greek yoghurt (acceptable in this phase), or nuts to temper their impact on your blood sugar. Or use them to garnish a salad – the oil in the dressing serves the same purpose. Melon with prosciutto is a classic fruit-and-protein combo.

MORE DAIRY OPTIONS

In addition to Phase 1 cheeses (pages 31–2) and additional dairy products and substitutes, your options now expand. Always select whole-milk or full-fat dairy products, including yoghurt. Low-fat dairy products are higher in carbs.

- Cottage cheese (not low-fat), creamed or curd style
- Ricotta cheese, made with whole milk
- Yoghurt or Greek yoghurt, natural whole milk, unsweetened
- Whole milk, fresh (limit to 4 tablespoons) or evaporated (limit to 2 tablespoons).

MAKE IT EASY

Flavoured yoghurts are full of sugar. Instead, add fresh or frozen fruit (unsweetened berries, cherries, or melon), unsweetened cocoa, instant coffee, or unsweetened coconut, plus a sprinkle of an acceptable sweetener, to natural yoghurt made with whole milk. The Greek type is lowest in carbs.

LEGUMES (PULSES)

Most legumes are sold dried or in tins, although a few, such as green soybeans (edamame) and baby lima beans, are usually sold fresh or frozen. (Green and wax beans are foundation vegetables, as are mangetout, meaning they are acceptable in Phase 1.) Avoid products such as baked beans made with added sugar. Hummus is a fine choice, but watch out for bean dips made with sugar or starches. You may choose to wait to reintroduce legumes until you move to Phase 3.

- Black beans (also called turtle beans)
- Black-eyed peas
- Broad beans
- Butter beans
- Chickpeas
- Edamame
- Haricot beans
- Hummus
- Kidney beans
- Peas, split
- Pinto beans
- Soybeans

TOMATO AND LEMON/LIME JUICE

In Phase 1 you could have 2 tablespoons lemon or lime juice; now you can have:

- 50 ml (2 fl oz) lemon or lime juice
- 125 ml (4 fl oz) tomato juice or tomato juice cocktail.

All other fruit and vegetable juices remain off-limits.

FOOLPROOF ADVICE TO STAY IN CONTROL

Understand that as you move through the phases and up the Carb Ladder, your objective is not to increase the amount of food you eat, but instead to introduce greater variety. In many cases this means that you'll be making substitutions rather than additions. To stay in control of your appetite as you reintroduce carb foods:

- Put aside certain foods in the morning, such as 20 pecan or walnut halves or 4 large strawberries, to incorporate into your accustomed Induction meals.
- Add sunflower seeds to salads rather than eating them out of hand.
- Swap fresh cheeses for the aged cheeses of Phase I.
- Treat berries and melon as garnishes – perhaps a couple of strawberries on a salad or a slice of melon wrapped in ham as part of your lunch.
- Top berries with Greek yoghurt instead of whipping cream.
- Stir a couple of tablespoons of plain Greek yoghurt into steamed spinach.
- Combine yoghurt with mayo when making egg or tuna salad.
- Stuff celery sticks with hummus instead of cream cheese.
- Have a small glass of tomato juice in lieu of sliced tomatoes with your breakfast eggs.
- Instead of radishes or red pepper slices, pair edamame with a piece of cheese as a snack.

ATKINS FOR VEGETARIANS

If you're a vegetarian, I recommend that you start Atkins in Phase 2 (Balancing), at 25–30 grams of Net Carbs a day so that you get sufficient protein. Most vegetarian sources of protein also contain carbs, unlike most animal products. Read the chapters on Induction, but include nuts and seeds from the start. The following protein products are acceptable, but check the Nutrition Information panel and the Atkins Carb Counter for Net Carb counts and serving sizes. Veggie burgers, for example, can vary dramatically in carb count, depending upon ingredients.

- Quorn cutlets, burgers, roast (unbreaded only)
- Tofu: firm, silken, or soft (not marinated)
- Tofu bacon, hot dogs, or sausage
- Tempeh (without grains)
- Seitan (available in health food shops and online)
- Shirataki soya noodles (available in Asian supermarkets and online)
- Veggie burgers, crumbles, or meatballs.

PHASE 2 LOW-CARB PRODUCTS

Although not part of the Carb Ladder, certain low-carb products can be introduced in this phase, including Atkins Endulge bars, Atkins low-carb pasta and Atkins Crunchy Muesli. You may also be able to have, in moderation, products such as low-carb bread, tortillas, wraps, or crisps with no more than 6 grams of Net Carbs per serving. Atkins cannot vouch for the carb counts or ingredients in other companies' products, so study the Nutrition Information panels and ingredients lists carefully to assess the Net Carb count and find any added sugar or other unacceptable ingredients. If any of these foods provoke cravings, stop eating them for the time being. For more details, see the Atkins Carb Counter.

WEEK-AT-A-GLANCE MEAL PLAN FOR WEEK 1 OF PHASE 2

As in Phase 1, you'll spread your carb intake across the day to keep your blood sugar on an even keel. You'll continue to enjoy the protein, foundation vegetables, and acceptable Phase 1 dairy products you've been eating, but you'll add nuts and/or seeds. To make this transition easy, we've modified the Week 1 Phase 1 meal plan to show you how to include about 5 grams of Net Carbs of nuts or seeds each day (shown in boldface italic type). Your daily intake should range from 23–27 grams of Net Carbs, averaging out to 25. As with earlier meal plans, feel free to modify this one to suit your preferences, substituting your own recipes or those in the section starting on page 211.

To update your shopping list, simply add the two items in boldface italics to your Phase 1 Week 1 shopping list. Also add any foods resulting from your modifications to the meal plan for this week.

PHASE 2 (BALANCING) WEEK 1

PROTEINS	DAIRY/CHEESE	VEGETABLES	CONDIMENTS/ NUTS	ATKINS PRODUCTS
Steak or Beef Burgers	Butter	Hass Avocados	Creamy Italian Dressing*	Atkins Bars
Chicken	Cheddar Cheese	Baby Spinach	Mayonnaise* or Tartare Sauce*	Atkins Shakes
Eggs	Mozzarella Cheese	Broccoli	Ranch Dressing*	Atkins Drinks
Ham or Pork Chops		Celery	Vinaigrette*	
Tinned Tuna or Fish Fillets		Lettuce/Salad Leaves	Extra-Virgin Olive Oil	
Bacon		Onions	*Almonds*	
Sausages		Red Peppers	*Walnuts*	
		Tomatoes		

*Select sauces and condiments without added sugar.

TO DRINK OR NOT TO DRINK? THAT IS THE QUESTION

Alcoholic beverages are permissible in Phase 2 (Balancing). But your body burns alcohol, just as it does carbohydrate and fat. In fact, it burns alcohol before fat and after blood sugar (from carbs). So drinking wine, beer, or spirits delays fat burning. Although white and brown spirits (whisky, rum, gin, vodka, etc.) contain no carbs, a 100-ml (3½-fl oz) serving of white, red, or dry dessert wine contains 1, 2, or 4 grams of carbs, respectively. A 30-ml (1-fl oz) serving of spirits or a glass of wine is not going to have a big impact on your daily carb tally, but beer is another story. A 350 ml (12 fl oz) can or bottle of most beer contains upwards of 13 grams of carbs. Low-carb or "lite" beers cut that to roughly 2.5 or 5.6 grams, respectively. Avoid wine coolers and conventional mixers, which are full of sugar. Fortunately, there are quite a few sugar-free mixers available. So should you drink once you reach OWL? That depends.

- Can you stop at one drink (for women) or two drinks (for men)?
- Are you willing to drink spirits neat, with soda water or with a sugar-free mixer?
- Can you moderate your intake of snacks such as salted peanuts or any other food when imbibing?

If the answer to any of these questions is no, you're probably better off waiting until you're closer to your goal weight to reintroduce alcohol.

CHEERS, SUGAR-FREE!

- Most cocktails present liquid trouble. A 100-ml (3½-fl oz) margarita, for example, racks up almost 14 grams of Net Carbs, and a piña colada more than 22 grams. But here's the good news. American Sweets sugar-free cocktail mixers (www.american-sweets.co.uk) make sugar-free mixers for various drinks. You may not find every option, but you'll be able to find mixers for a bloody Mary, daiquiri, mai tai, margarita, cranberry or sour apple martini, mojito, mudslide, piña colada, and sweet and sour.

Atkins Phase 2 (Balancing) Meal Plan at 25 g NC/day: Week 1

	MONDAY	TUESDAY	WEDNESDAY	THURSDAY
BREAKFAST	2 eggs 40 g chopped onion 1 tsp olive oil 30 g Cheddar cheese 60 g bacon or sausage Net Carbs: 4.1 g; FV: 3.1 g	Atkins Advantage Chocolate Hazelnut Bar *25 almonds* Net Carbs: 5.7 g; FV: 0 g	2 eggs 60–115 g ham 1 tbsp olive oil 3 tbsp chopped onion 1 small tomato Net Carbs: 5.6 g; FV: 4.8 g	115–175 g steak or beefburger 1 tsp olive oil 90 g chopped pepper 40 g chopped onion 60 g Cheddar cheese Net Carbs: 6 g; FV: 5.3 g
SNACK	Atkins Day Break Almond Cranberry Bar *25 almonds* Net Carbs: 6.7 g; FV: 0 g	1 small tomato 30 g Cheddar cheese Net Carbs: 2.6 g; FV: 2.5 g	Atkins Day Break Cappuccino Nut Bar *10 walnut halves* Net Carbs: 4.9 g; FV: 0 g	2 celery sticks 30 g mozzarella cheese Net Carbs: 2.2 g; FV: 2 g
LUNCH	115–175 g ham or pork chop 1 small tomato 30 g baby spinach 2 tbsp Vinaigrette* Net Carbs: 4.3 g; FV: 4 g	115–175 g chicken 1 small tomato 55 g mixed lettuce ½ avocado 2 tbsp Ranch Dressing* 20 almonds Net Carbs: 8.1 g; FV: 5.1 g	115–175 g steak or beefburger 110 g mixed lettuce ½ avocado 2 tbsp Vinaigrette* Net Carbs: 4.3 g; FV: 4 g	Atkins Advantage Chocolate Decadence Bar *15 walnut halves* Net Carbs: 4.1 g; FV: 0 g
SNACK	Atkins Advantage Café Royal RTD *20 almonds* Net Carbs: 3.6 g; FV: 0 g	1 celery stick 30 g Cheddar cheese Net Carbs: 1.4 g; FV: 1 g	1 small tomato 30 g Cheddar cheese *25 almonds* Net Carbs: 5.5 g; FV: 2.5 g	1 small tomato 2 tbsp Vinaigrette* *25 almonds* Net Carbs: 5.7 g; FV: 2.5 g
DINNER	115–175 g tinned tuna or fish fillet 110 g mixed lettuce ½ avocado 2 tbsp Vinaigrette* 90 g broccoli florets Net Carbs: 6 g; FV: 5.6 g	115–175 g steak or beefburger ½ medium pepper ⅓ small onion 55 g mixed lettuce 2 tbsp Ranch Dressing* Net Carbs: 6.3 g; FV: 5.5 g	115–175 g chicken 90 g broccoli florets 110 g mixed lettuce 2 tbsp Creamy Italian Dressing* Net Carbs: 4.5 g; FV: 4.3 g	115–175 g chicken 60 g baby spinach 45 g sliced pepper 1 small tomato 2 tbsp Ranch Dressing* Net Carbs: 6.5 g; FV: 5.8 g
	Total Net Carbs: 24.7 g Total Net Carbs from FV: 12.7 g	Total Net Carbs: 24.1 g Total Net Carbs from FV: 14.1 g	Total Net Carbs: 24.8 g Total Net Carbs from FV: 15.6 g	Total Net Carbs: 24.5 g Total Net Carbs from FV: 15.6 g

FRIDAY	SATURDAY	SUNDAY
60 g baby spinach	2 eggs	2 eggs
1 tbsp olive oil	60 g bacon or sausage	60 g baby spinach
1 small tomato	1 small tomato	1 tsp olive oil
½ avocado		½ pepper
30 g Cheddar cheese		60 g cheese
Net Carbs: 6.8 g; FV: 6.8 g	Net Carbs: 4.5 g; FV: 2.5 g	Net Carbs: 6.4 g; FV: 5.3 g
Atkins Day Break Strawberry Yoghurt RTD	New Atkins Day Break Strawberry Crisp Bar	1 celery stick
	25 almonds	30 g Cheddar cheese
Net Carbs: 3 g; FV: 0 g	Net Carbs: 5.8 g; FV: 0 g	Net Carbs: 1.4 g; FV: 1 g
115–175 g chicken	115–175 g tinned tuna or fish fillet	Atkins Advantage Dark Chocolate Crunch Bar
110 g mixed lettuce	2 tbsp mayonnaise or tartare	*20 walnut halves*
45 g sliced pepper	sauce*	
2 tbsp Creamy Italian Dressing*	1 celery stick	
	45 g chopped pepper	
	1 small tomato	
	15 walnut halves	
Net Carbs: 4.8 g; FV: 4.5 g	Net Carbs: 7.1 g; FV: 5 g	Net Carbs: 6.5 g; FV: 0 g
Atkins Advantage Milk Chocolate RTD	2 celery sticks	90 g chopped pepper
25 almonds	2½ tbsp Creamy Italian Dressing*	2 tbsp Ranch Dressing*
		25 almonds
Net Carbs: 4.1 g; FV: 0 g	Net Carbs: 2.2 g; FV: 2 g	Net Carbs: 5.5 g; FV: 2.2 g
115–175 g ham or pork chop	115–175 g steak or beef burger	175 g chicken
90 g broccoli	30 g Cheddar cheese	90 g broccoli
55 g mixed lettuce	1 small tomato	1 tsp olive oil
1 small tomato	½ avocado	55 g mixed lettuce
2 tbsp Creamy Italian Dressing*	½ small onion	½ avocado
10 walnut halves		2 tbsp Vinaigrette*
Net Carbs: 7 g; FV: 5.4 g	Net Carbs: 6.7 g; FV: 6.5 g	Net Carbs: 4.6 g; FV: 4.2 g
Total Net Carbs: 25.7 g	Total Net Carbs: 26.3 g	Total Net Carbs: 24.4 g
Total Net Carbs from FV: 16.7g	Total Net Carbs from FV: 16 g	Total Net Carbs from FV: 12.7 g

THE SCOOP ON SUGAR: PRIME OFFENDERS

Added sugars are found in countless common foods. Here's the (not so) skinny on a few that you may have been eating and drinking before you began Atkins, starting with those in which you wouldn't expect to find sugar and ending with those in which it's a key ingredient. Prepare to be astounded!

FOOD	SERVING	SUGAR CONTENT
Jif Creamy Peanut Butter	2 tablespoons	3 grams
Kikkoman Seasoned Rice Vinegar	1 tablespoon	4 grams
Burger King BBQ Dip	1 packet	6.3 grams
Kellogg's Nutri-grain Oat & Choc Chip Bar	1 bar	12 grams
Heinz Baked Beans	200 g	10.3 grams
Baxter's Cream of Tomato Soup	200 g	10.2 grams
Glaceau Vitamin C Water	100 ml	3 grams
Go Ahead Crispy Forest Fruits	1 slice	4.9 grams
Lee Kum Kee Hoisin Sauce	42 g	20.2 grams
Victoria Sponge Mix	42 g	12.5 grams
7UP Lemon & Lime	100 ml	11.2 grams
McDonald's Crunchy McFlurry	per serving	46 grams
Activia Strawberry Yoghurt	125 g	16.8 grams
Ocean Spray Cranberry Juice	100 ml	13.8 grams
Lyle's Golden Syrup	100 ml	80.5 grams

FREQUENTLY ASKED QUESTIONS

Q. How long do I need to continue with salty stock or another salt source?

A. As long as you're no longer having symptoms of dehydration or electrolyte imbalance such as fatigue, dizziness on standing, leg cramps, or constipation, you can stop, regardless of whether you stay in Phase 1 or move on to Phase 2. Continue to salt your food normally and drink plenty of fluids. Feel free to continue with the stock if you find it filling and soothing.

Q. I've had trouble moving from weight loss to weight maintenance in the past. How can I keep the weight off this time?
A. If you previously lost all your excess weight in Phase 1 before trying to maintain your new weight, I strongly suggest you follow the Slow and Steady path this time. In Chapter 8, you'll find techniques to help you stay in control over the long term.

Q. If I miss berries more than nuts and seeds, can I add them back first?
A. As long as you can control your portions and proceed with caution, you can reorder the introduction of Phase 2 (Balancing) acceptable foods on the Carb Ladder. However, nuts and seeds are full of protein and fat, making them more satiating than berries, although both are relatively low in carbs.

Q. If I'm extremely overweight, is it safe to exercise?
A. Yes, in general, but consult with your GP first. Once you have the go-ahead, your best bets are activities that don't stress your joints, such as chair exercises, swimming, pedalling a reclining stationary bike, and water exercises. Walking and bike riding are also good choices.

Q. How can I determine the carb count of a restaurant meal?
A. Most casual dining and fast-food chains offer nutritional data online, so you can decide ahead of time what to order. Some apps allow you to subtract or add certain items such as a roll, mustard, or tomato on a burger, for example, or see the impact of grilled chicken with and without fries. Nonetheless, you're often on your own, which is where the Atkins mobile app and Atkins Carb Counter come to the rescue.

In the next chapter, we'll discuss how to gradually move up the Carb Ladder, reintroducing more variety and more grams of Net Carbs back into your meals as you continue to slim down. This is all part of finding your personal carb balance. We'll also probe how to troubleshoot a weight-loss plateau and other issues. But before that, let me introduce you to Heather H., whose embarrassment over her size had made her a virtual hermit. Before embarking on Atkins, she did her homework to make sure she knew how to do it correctly. And she has, as her impressive results make clear.

PREPARATION IS THE SECRET TO SUCCESS

VITAL STATS

Daily Net Carb intake:
   20 grams
Age: 43
Height: 166 cm (5 ft 5½ in)

Before weight: 148 kg
   (23 st 5 lb)
After weight: 90 kg (14 st)
Lost: 58 kg (135 lb)

Heather H. had spent her thirties hiding from life, too embarrassed to go out in public. During that time the Mountain Home, Arkansas resident had developed Type 2 diabetes, along with diabetic kidney disease, high cholesterol, and severe sleep apnoea. Although Heather had tried other diets, including Atkins, without success, the idea of facing her forties in the same sorry shape was unacceptable. She was ready to enjoy life, and she knew Atkins was the key that would open that door. Heather relates her inspiring tale.

I had always been a big girl, but I was in a terrible marriage and really let myself go. My endocrinologist said that, although my kidney disease was at an early stage, if I didn't get in shape I could lose one or more limbs. The only thing that was going well was my work. I work at home developing software for public education. I had done Atkins in 2003 and lost 27 kg (60 lb), but after having a miscarriage, I regained the weight. What did I eat? The better question is what didn't I eat. I'd have potatoes, bread, sweets, biscuits, and all the other things that were wrong for my metabolism. I was never a moody eater and I'd eat regularly, but my meals were two or three times as large as a normal meal.

When I was ready to lose the weight once and for all, I took my time. I spent two months reading *The New Atkins for a New You*, finding low-carb recipes, and planning menus. I also started preparing for a total life change. I knew that once I started I would remain on Atkins forever. Potatoes, pasta, and pastries are just not an option for my body. I also started walking for 30–40 minutes every day around the neighbourhood.

I began Atkins in May 2011, the day after my 41st birthday. My family was wonderfully supportive. Within six months I'd lost 43 kg (95 lb), my blood-sugar levels were excellent, my cholesterol had improved, and I am no longer classified as having diabetic kidney disease. I'm also able to sleep again without the aid of the CPAP (continuous positive airway pressure) mask. The weight comes off more slowly now, but I've lost 58 kg (135 lb) and am working towards my goal weight of 78.5 kg (12 st 5 lb).

I'm totally into Atkins, but I'm not really into cooking. And I'm not really a breakfast person, so I usually have an Atkins bar – my favourites are the Peanut Butter Fudge and the brownies – or a shake instead. I always read labels, and believe me, sugar is everywhere. I have the Atkins Carb Counter app on my smartphone, which really helps me, especially when I'm eating at a new place. I also have menus from all over for takeaways. As I said, I like to be prepared!

How much I weigh is not as much of an issue to me as my health and how I feel. Still, I've gone from wearing UK oversize 36–38 (US oversize 6X) jeans to UK size 14 (US size 12). Yay! It feels so nice to be able to breathe, to tie my shoelaces, to get into a car and not have to push the seat all the way back to fit in. Even little things like riding a bike and being able to sit comfortably in a cinema or restaurant are simply amazing! I've regained my confidence and am no longer ashamed to be seen in public.

Losing weight helped me make the decision to divorce my husband. Dating again is strange but fun. My daughter is so proud of me, and I'm proud to be a role model for her. For the first time in 12 years I really want to get out and do things. I feel great and I want to see the world – and the world to see me!

MAKE IT EASY

Be sure there's always plenty of food in the house by cooking up a big batch, so when you get hungry, you aren't tempted to eat the wrong thing. Peanuts are my favourite snack. Just be sure to portion them out in 30 g (1 oz) bags. *–HH*

CHAPTER 6

BEGIN TO FIND YOUR PERSONAL CARB BALANCE

I'll bet you're looking forward to savouring strawberries, blueberries, melon, cottage cheese, yoghurt, and more, along with the nuts and seeds you've probably already reintroduced. If you've chosen to take the Slow and Steady path by starting to climb the Carb Ladder, you'll begin to explore these and other foods that will add delicious variety to your meals. (If you've chosen the Fast Track, see "Remaining in Phase 1 – for Now", page 109.) Patience is essential for an easy transition from Phase 1 (Kick-Start) to Phase 2 (Balancing).

Instead of adding these foods all at once, start with the berries and other acceptable fruits listed on page 93, introducing them one by one. Wait a couple of days at the very least after you reintroduce blueberries, for example, before trying strawberries or cantaloupe, to gauge your response. If one fruit doesn't cause cravings or stimulate your appetite for more, try another. Then, and only then, move on to the dairy products listed on page 94, at the same time increasing your daily Net Carb intake by 5 grams. By slowly exploring greater flexibility and freedom of choice as you move up the Carb Ladder, you can ease from one phase to the next while continuing to experience the empowering sense of control to which you've become accustomed. You'll use this latitude to begin the process of finding your personal carb balance, the amount and variety of carb foods you can consume while continuing to lose weight, feel great, and remain in control of your appetite. If you're on the Slow and Steady path, you're likely to spend a significant amount of time and lose most of your excess weight in Phase 2. Depending on how sensitive you are to carbs and how much weight you want to lose, this could take anywhere from several weeks to a number of months. But regardless of the amount of time it takes, follow the rungs of the Carb Ladder and the suggestions below to ease the process.

WHAT TO EXPECT IN PHASE 2

Initially Phase 2 (Balancing) of the New Atkins is very similar to Phase 1 (Kick-Start). You take the first baby step as you increase to 25 daily grams of Net Carbs. As long as you anticipate certain situations, you'll retain that sense of control over your appetite and intake, although you may have to make some mid-course corrections. You'll likely experience several things in this phase.

- *The pace of your weight loss may slow.* Unless you have lots of weight to shed, the rapid weight loss that you may have experienced in the initial phase usually slows down. This may not happen immediately, but when it eventually does, be prepared, understand that it's perfectly normal, and adjust your expectations accordingly. After all, as you slim down, each banished pound represents a greater percentage of your remaining weight. And weight is only one measure of your success. Equally important are your energy levels and mood.
- *Your hunger level may increase.* As you add more carbs and reintroduce certain foods you may find yourself hungrier than you were in Induction. This makes it all the more important that you do not go too long between meals and snacks, and continue to eat the recommended amounts of protein and fat.
- *Cravings may return.* After thinking you were permanently rid of the cravings that almost miraculously disappeared in your weeks in Induction, you may find that it's hard to stop eating certain foods or they make you crave other carb foods. We'll discuss how to deal with cravings below.
- *You may experience weight-loss plateaux.* This can happen at any time but is increasingly likely the longer you spend losing weight. Your body has its own internal logic, as you'll learn in "A Plateau Calls for Patience", page 118.

REMAINING IN PHASE 1 – FOR NOW

If you've decided to stay at 20 grams of Net Carbs for the time being but have added nuts and seeds, read this chapter to learn what to expect when the time comes to move to Phase 2. Again, you should do so no later than when you're 7 kg (15 lb) from your goal weight. On page 117, I'll address the issue of weight-loss plateaux while you're still in Phase 1. Remember, you can move to Phase 2 at any time if you desire more variety in your carb choices.

EVALUATE YOUR FIRST WEEK IN PHASE 2

If you followed the guidelines in the previous chapter (pages 46–7) to the letter, you probably found your first week smooth sailing. However, if you overdid things – perhaps overindulging in peanuts, for example – you may need to rein in your enthusiasm. Also, if you have a very low tolerance for carbs, even the slight increase to 25 daily grams of Net Carbs might have slowed down weight loss. Let's try to tease out whether all is well or you need to make a minor adjustment. Start out with your usual weekly weigh-in and measurements. Then answer these questions.

- *Did you lose any weight?* If so, and if you can say with certainty that you're doing Phase 2 (Balancing) properly, relax. If the number on the scale didn't represent as great a loss as the week before, understand that you cannot expect to lose the same amount of weight week after week, particularly once you leave the initial phase of Atkins.
- *Did you lose girth?* Once again, girth often disappears before weight and is a good indicator that you're moving in the right direction.
- *Did you lose neither weight nor girth?* If so, review the guidelines to be sure that you're doing everything correctly and not over-doing serving sizes.
- *Are you experiencing cravings?* If any food causes cravings, stop eating it for several days before trying to reintroduce it. If you find it hard to stop with a few almonds, or that an hour after you eat a small portion of blueberries you're just dying for more, you need to act – fast. Note these events in your journal, along

with whether (and how) you were able to control the cravings. Perhaps you ate those berries "naked" the first time before realising you're better off serving them with whipped cream or nuts. Or you dug into a supersized container of almonds instead of putting 30 g (1 oz) into a small resealable bag.

- *Are you hungrier than you were in Induction?* Stay alert to hunger signals; if and when they hit, have a low-carb snack. Or eat your next meal a little earlier than you might otherwise.

MOVING TO WEEK 2 OF PHASE 2

Your results in the first week will determine your actions as you move into Week 2. If you lost weight and girth and weren't plagued anew with cravings and undue hunger, you may feel comfortable moving up to 30 grams of daily Net Carbs after just a week. If you wish, you can also move up one rung on the Carb Ladder (see page 14) and begin eating berries, cherries, and most kinds of melon. (See the meal plan on pages 112–13.) However, if your weight loss slowed and you found it more difficult to stay in control, you're better off remaining at 25 grams of Net Carbs without going up another rung on the Carb Ladder. Instead, for variety, you could play with introducing other nuts and/or seeds. This will give your system time to adapt to these foods and the slightly higher carb intake of OWL.

Don't regard a slowdown in your weekly weight loss as a defeat, and don't rush back to the security of Phase 1 (Kick-Start). Depending on the efficiency of your fat-burning engine, you may be able to climb the Carb Ladder quickly and increase your daily Net Carb intake every week or so, or you may need to proceed much more slowly. Small moves enable you to remain in control. Tailor your journey based on your weekly weight and girth loss and your response to foods on different steps of the ladder.

WEEK-AT-A-GLANCE MEAL PLAN AT 30 GRAMS OF NET CARBS

The meal plan on pages 112–13 represents the second step up the Carb Ladder (see page 14). You'll continue to enjoy the Phase 1 (Kick-Start) foods, as well as the nuts and/or seeds you've recently added. The only difference is that you'll add about 5 grams of Net

Carbs from the berries and other low-carb fruits listed on page 93. We've again modified the original meal plan to show how to include them. See the simple suggestions indicated in **boldface italics** in the meal plan on pages 112–13 for how to add these foods. (They are also in **boldface italic** type on the shopping list below.) Additions are small and incremental, ensuring that changes take place slowly, which moderates any impact on your blood-sugar levels. Feel free to substitute other Phase 2 fruits for the items listed, using the Atkins Carb Counter to check their carb counts.

PHASE 2 (BALANCING) WEEK 2

PROTEINS	DAIRY/CHEESES	VEGETABLES	CONDIMENTS/ NUTS	ATKINS PRODUCTS/ FRUIT
Steak or Beef Burgers	Butter	Hass Avocados	Creamy Italian Dressing*	Atkins Bars
Chicken	Cheddar Cheese	Baby Spinach	Mayonnaise* or Tartare Sauce*	Atkins Shakes
Eggs	Mozzarella Cheese	Broccoli	Ranch Dressing*	Atkins Low Carb Pasta
Ham or Pork Chops		Celery	Vinaigrette*	**Strawberries**
Tinned Tuna or Fish Fillets		Lettuce/Salad Leaves	Extra-Virgin Olive Oil	**Cantaloupe**
Bacon or Sausages		Onions	Almonds	**Raspberries**
		Red Peppers	Walnuts	
		Tomatoes		

*Select sauces and condiments without added sugar.

Atkins Phase 2 (Balancing) Meal Plan at 30 g NC/day

	MONDAY	TUESDAY	WEDNESDAY	THURSDAY

BREAKFAST	2 eggs
	40 g chopped onion
	1 tsp olive oil
	30 g Cheddar cheese
	60 g bacon or sausage
	
	Net Carbs: 4.1 g; FV: 3.1 g
		Atkins Advantage
		  Chocolate Hazelnut
		  Crunch Bar
		25 almonds
		5 large strawberries
		
		Net Carbs: 10.9 g; FV: 0 g
			2 eggs
			60–115 g ham
			1 tbsp olive oil
			3 tbsp chopped onion
			1 small tomato
			50 g cantaloupe cubes
			Net Carbs: 9.5 g; FV: 4.8 g
				115–175 g steak or beefburger
				1 tsp olive oil
				90 g chopped pepper
				40 g chopped onion
				60 g Cheddar cheese
				
				Net Carbs: 6 g; FV: 5.3 g

SNACK	Atkins Day Break Almond
	  Cranberry Bar
	25 almonds
	
	Net Carbs: 6.7 g; FV: 0 g
		1 small tomato
		30 g Cheddar cheese
		
		Net Carbs: 2.6 g; FV: 2.5 g
			Atkins Day Break
			  Cappuccino Nut Bar
			10 walnut halves
			
			Net Carbs: 4.9 g; FV: 0 g
				2 celery sticks
				30 g mozzarella cheese
				
				Net Carbs: 2.2 g; FV: 2 g

LUNCH	115–175 g ham or pork
	  chop
	1 small tomato
	30 g baby spinach
	2 tbsp Vinaigrette*
	5 large strawberries
	Net Carbs: 9.4 g; FV: 4 g
		115–175 g chicken
		1 small tomato
		55 g mixed lettuce
		½ avocado
		2 tbsp Ranch Dressing*
		20 almonds
		Net Carbs: 8.1 g; FV: 5.1 g
			115–175 g steak or
			  beefburger
			110 g mixed lettuce
			½ avocado
			2 tbsp Vinaigrette*
			
			Net Carbs: 4.3 g; FV: 4 g
				Atkins Advantage Chocolate
				  Decadence Bar
				15 walnut halves
				
				Net Carbs: 4.1 g; FV: 0 g

SNACK	Atkins Advantage Café Royal RTD 20 almonds Net Carbs: 3.6 g; FV: 0 g	1 celery stick 30 g Cheddar cheese Net Carbs: 1.4 g; FV: 1 g	1 small tomato 30 g Cheddar cheese 25 almonds Net Carbs: 5.5 g; FV: 2.5 g	1 small tomato 2 tbsp Vinaigrette* 25 almonds Net Carbs: 5.7 g; FV: 2.5 g

DINNER	115–175 g tinned tuna or
	  fish fillet
	110 g mixed lettuce
	½ avocado
	2 tbsp Vinaigrette*
	90 g broccoli florets
	Net Carbs: 6 g; FV: 5.6 g
		115–175 g steak or
		  beefburger
		½ medium pepper
		⅓ small onion
		55 g mixed lettuce
		2 tbsp Ranch Dressing*
		Net Carbs: 6.3 g; FV: 5.5 g
			115–175 g chicken
			90 g broccoli florets
			110 g mixed lettuce
			2 tbsp Creamy Italian
			  Dressing*
			
			Net Carbs: 4.5 g; FV: 4.3 g
				115–175 g chicken
				60 g baby spinach
				45 g sliced pepper
				1 small tomato
				2 tbsp Ranch Dressing
				80 g cantaloupe cubes
				Net Carbs: 12.3 g; FV: 5.8 g

	Total Net Carbs: 29.8 g
	Total Net Carbs from FV:
	  12.7 g
		Total Net Carbs: 29.3 g
		Total Net Carbs from FV:
		  14.1 g
			Total Net Carbs: 28.7 g
			Total Net Carbs from FV:
			  15.6 g
				Total Net Carbs: 30.3 g
				Total Net Carbs from FV:
				  15.6 g

BEGIN TO FIND YOUR PERSONAL CARB BALANCE

FRIDAY	SATURDAY	SUNDAY
60 g baby spinach 1 tbsp olive oil 1 small tomato ½ avocado 30 g Cheddar cheese	2 eggs 60 g bacon or sausage 1 small tomato *60 g raspberries*	2 eggs 60 g baby spinach 1 tsp olive oil ½ pepper 60 g Cheddar cheese *50 g cantaloupe cubes*
Net Carbs: 6.8 g; FV: 6.8 g	Net Carbs: 7.8 g; FV: 2.5 g	Net Carbs: 10.3 g; FV: 5.3 g
Atkins Day Break Strawberry Yoghurt RTD *5 large strawberries*	Atkins Day Break Strawberry Crisp Bar 25 almonds	1 celery stick 30 g Cheddar cheese
Net Carbs: 8.1 g; FV: 0 g	Net Carbs: 5.8 g; FV: 0 g	Net Carbs: 1.4 g; FV: 1 g
115–175 g chicken 110 g mixed greens 45 g sliced pepper 2 tbsp Creamy Italian Dressing*	115–175 g tinned tuna or fish fillet 2 tbsp mayonnaise or tartare sauce* 1 celery stick 45 g chopped pepper 1 small tomato 15 walnut halves	Atkins Advantage Dark Chocolate Crunch Bar 20 walnut halves *60 g raspberries*
Net Carbs: 4.8 g; FV: 4.5 g	Net Carbs: 7.1 g; FV: 5 g	Net Carbs: 9.9 g; FV: 0 g
Atkins Advantage Milk Chocolate RTD 25 almonds *5 large strawberries*	2 celery sticks 2½ tbsp Creamy Italian Dressing*	90 g chopped pepper 2 tbsp Ranch Dressing* 25 almonds
Net Carbs: 9.3 g; FV: 0 g	Net Carbs: 2.2 g; FV: 2 g	Net Carbs: 5.5 g; FV: 2.2 g
115–175 g ham or pork chop 90 g broccoli 55 g mixed lettuce 1 small tomato 2 tbsp Creamy Italian Dressing* 10 walnut halves	115–175 g steak or beef burger 30 g Cheddar cheese 1 small tomato ½ avocado ½ small onion	175 g chicken 90 g broccoli 1 tsp olive oil 55 g mixed lettuce ½ avocado 2 tbsp Vinaigrette*
Net Carbs: 7 g; FV: 5.4 g	Net Carbs: 6.7 g; FV: 6.5 g	Net Carbs: 4.6 g; FV: 4.2 g
Total Net Carbs: 36 g Total Net Carbs from FV: 12.4 g	Total Net Carbs: 29.6 g Total Net Carbs from FV: 16 g	Total Net Carbs: 31.7 g Total Net Carbs from FV: 12.7 g

WEEK 3 AND BEYOND IN PHASE 2

Assuming that you've already added nuts and seeds and then berries and the like, as discussed previously, your next move will be to introduce foods on the next rung of the Carb Ladder. These additional dairy products include natural yoghurt or Greek yoghurt (made with whole milk, not the flavoured or low-fat kind), cottage cheese, and ricotta. You can also have small portions of whole milk. In some cases, you'll be swapping other foods (replacing Cheddar cheese, for example, with yoghurt) to keep carbs in line. After additional dairy products come legumes, and finally tomato and tomato juice cocktail, as well as more lemon and/or lime juice. (See page 14 to review these rungs of the Carb Ladder.) To modify the earlier meal plans to make them suitable for 35, 40, and 45 grams of Net Carbs, follow these guidelines:

Additional dairy rung: Reintroduce these foods in portions of roughly 5 grams of Net Carbs. For example:

85 g (3 oz) cottage cheese	4.1 grams Net Carbs
85 g (3 oz) ricotta cheese	4 grams Net Carbs
50 ml (2 fl oz) buttermilk	3.3 grams Net Carbs
50 ml (2 fl oz) whole milk	2.9 grams Net Carbs
125 g (4½ oz) Greek yoghurt (plain, unsweetened, made with whole milk)	4.5 grams Net Carbs
125 g (4½ oz) yoghurt (plain, unsweetened, made with whole milk)	5.3 grams Net Carbs

Legumes rung: Reintroduce these foods in portions of roughly 5 grams of Net Carbs. For example:

2 tablespoons cooked chickpeas	5.5 grams Net Carbs
20 g (¾ oz) cooked lentils	4 grams Net Carbs
2 tablespoons cooked haricot beans	5 grams Net Carbs
20 g (¾ oz) cooked split green peas	6.3 grams Net Carbs
40 g (1½ oz) shelled edamame (green soybeans)	3 grams Net Carbs
3 tablespoons black bean dip	4.5 grams Net Carbs
3 tablespoons hummus	4.5 grams Net Carbs

Tomato and lemon/lime juice rung: Reintroduce these foods in portions of roughly 5 grams of Net Carbs. You can also increase lemon or lime juice from 2 to 4 tablespoons a day.

4 tablespoons lemon juice	4 grams Net Carbs
4 tablespoons lime juice	4.8 grams Net Carbs
125 ml (4 fl oz) tomato juice	4.0 grams Net Carbs
125 ml (4 fl oz) tomato-vegetable juice cocktail	4.5 grams Net Carbs

Check the Atkins Carb Counter for other options.

However, as you seek your threshold for carb intake while continuing to shed weight, known as your carb balance, your daily Net Carb intake may level off well before you move to Phase 3 (Fine-Tuning). If you have a low-carb tolerance, you may choose to experiment by adding some or all of these foods without increasing your daily carb intake or by doing so very slowly.

QUICK PHASE 2 SNACKS

One way to shift into Ongoing Weight Loss is to keep your meals similar to those you ate in Phase 1, but now have snacks that incorporate Phase 2 foods. All Atkins bars and shakes are now acceptable, and you can certainly continue to have your favourites coded for Phase 1. Following are some other snacks you can put together in minutes if you have the ingredients in the fridge and or store cupboard. They're also portable. Pop them in an insulated bag with a freezer pack and take them to work or wherever. .

- Cottage cheese and berries
- Hummus with radishes or jicama sticks
- Celery sticks stuffed with almond or peanut butter
- Tomato juice with a slice of Cheddar cheese
- Greek yoghurt, blueberries, and a packet of sweetener
- Greek yoghurt mixed with no-sugar-added salsa, with soya chips
- Sliced avocado on a small low-carb pitta bread
- Chopped almonds mixed with half an Atkins bar cut into cubes
- Prosciutto wrapped around cantaloupe slices
- Provolone wrapped around honeydew melon slices

- Small low-carb tortilla with black bean dip and a tomato slice
- Cooked and shelled edamame drizzled with olive oil.

FIND YOUR PERSONAL CARB BALANCE

In Phase 1 (Kick-Start), you, your significant other, your boss, and your great-aunt Hilda can all eat the same amount of carbs and a fixed number of foods and pretty reliably shave off some excess weight. It's the rare individual who doesn't convert to burning primarily fat in the first week of Atkins. Phase 2 (Balancing) is a different story. Whether you're a fast loser or slow loser, in this phase you'll get to grips with your own metabolism. This understanding will be invaluable as you move towards a permanent way of eating.

There's tremendous variation in how many carbs individuals can consume while continuing to lose weight. (The same applies to maintaining weight, as we'll discuss in Chapter 8.) An active young man might be able to put away 70 grams of Net Carbs a day (or even more) and keep shedding weight. Meanwhile, a sedentary menopausal woman might hover around 40 grams or even less. Once you understand how sensitive your metabolism is to carbs in general and to certain foods in particular, you'll be armed with the information you need to tailor your progress up the Carb Ladder accordingly. Once more, your personal carb balance is the number of grams of Net Carbs you can consume while continuing to lose weight, feel good, and remain in control of your appetite. This number usually rises as you get closer to your goal.

TROUBLESHOOTING

As you continue to move up the Carb Ladder slowly but deliberately, your weight loss will slow and almost certainly not proceed like clockwork.

Both are normal. A loss of 1–1.5 kg (2–3 lb) a week might be a reasonable expectation for your age, weight, and other factors. However, some weeks you may pare off just a single pound or so, or even a big fat zero. Bottom line: be patient. If your weight loss stalls for several weeks, you may have exceeded your carb tolerance or you may have hit a plateau. How can you tell the difference? And what do you do to reignite fat burning? Let's start with the second question.

STALLED? WHAT'S THE PROBLEM?

Before you panic and jump to the conclusion that you'll never lose another pound or that you'll never get above, say, 45 grams of Net Carbs a day, ask yourself these questions.

- Are you counting (not estimating) grams of Net Carbs?
- Are you eating any inappropriate foods?
- Are you supersizing portions?
- Are you overdoing it with berries and/or low-carb products?
- Are you finding certain foods you can't eat in moderation?
- Are you adding additional food, meaning that you're eating more, rather than swapping out other foods (edamame for green beans, for example) to maintain the amount of food?
- Are you eating more than 175 g (6 oz) of protein at each meal?
- Have you added all Phase 2 acceptable foods at the same time?
- Have you started drinking wine or beer or using sugar-filled mixers?

Assuming that these queries merit some yes responses, it's time to make one or more modifications to get back on track.

- *Write it down.* Carb creep is all too common as you start to re-introduce certain foods. Enter your food choices, amounts, and Net Carb counts in your journal. You may well be consuming more carbs than you think you are.
- *Play hide and seek.* Look for carbs you may have neglected to count, such as in cream, lemon juice, and even acceptable sweeteners (reminder: count 1 gram of Net Carbs per packet). Also be vigilant about reading labels to ferret out hidden carbs in sauces, condiments, and other processed foods.

- *Abstain for now.* Drinking alcohol could be interfering with fat burning. Eliminate it, as well as any trigger foods.
- *Check your calories.* Although there's no need to count calories on a daily basis, a woman consuming more than 1,800 calories or a man consuming more than 2,200 may simply be eating too much.

If you're not actually on a plateau, you should see weight loss resume once you make the appropriate modifications.

A PLATEAU CALLS FOR PATIENCE

A plateau is defined as an inexplicable pause in weight loss for one month or longer that's not the result of dietary misdemeanours or lifestyle changes. It can happen at any time after you shed the first "easy" pounds, but it is increasingly likely as you approach your goal weight. For inexplicable reasons, your body simply slows down and "refuses" to lose any more weight for a while. Infuriating? Of course. Permanent? Fortunately not. A plateau usually yields to certain strategies, including temporarily reducing your daily carb intake. If you're at, say, 35 grams of Net Carbs a day and hit a plateau, you can cut back by 10 grams and likely some excess pounds will budge. You might even need to go down another 5 grams to 20 grams, which will almost certainly reboot weight loss. Once you're losing again, you can gradually start to increase the carbs.

One possibility is that you've stumbled upon your carb tolerance level without realising it. If cutting back on carbs doesn't do the trick, pretty much the only thing to do is wait out the plateau, although adding regular physical activity if you haven't already done so may also bust it. It will certainly help you maintain your weight and handle the stress the plateau occasions. (See "Nowhere to Go," opposite, if you plateau while following the Fast Track.)

Although it sounds counterintuitive, some people have found that slightly increasing their carb intake or adding a new acceptable food kick-starts weight loss again. Patience is definitely a virtue when it comes to a plateau. As you'll remember from Charity W.'s story (page 40), she waited out an eight-week period of no weight loss!

NOWHERE TO GO

If you're following the Fast Track by remaining in Phase 1, busting a plateau is challenging. When you're consuming just 20 daily grams of Net Carbs for an extended period of time, it may be tempting to drop below 20 grams a day, but it's not healthy to sacrifice foundation vegetables to do so. You simply have to hang in there. Moreover, overly restricting choices in Phase 1 can make the programme too difficult for the long haul.

IDENTIFY AND AVOID TRIGGER FOODS

If you can't seem to eat just a few nuts, you already know what a trigger food is: it's any food, whether an acceptable one such as nuts or an unacceptable one such as chocolate chip cookies, that you can't eat in moderate portions and which may make you hungry for other foods as well. Once you have one (or a handful), you can't stop eating until the box or bag or jar is empty. The best way to deal with unacceptable trigger foods is to banish them from the house if possible. With Atkins-friendly foods such as peanuts, measure out portions ahead of time to avoid overeating.

The urge to binge is a clear indicator that you may have exceeded your carb threshold. If you're eating too many carbs, fat burning ceases and with it the empowerment of appetite suppression. Bingeing isn't just a matter of eating more carbs than you should; it's being totally out of control, often as a result of eating a trigger food. Eating a second 30 g (1 oz) bag of almonds is an indiscretion; snarfing down a carton of rocky road ice cream is a binge. The only solution to such overindulgence is to stop it before it occurs.

In addition to not going too long between meals, always having acceptable foods in the house, and not shopping while you're hungry, these tips should help head off the urge to binge:

- Call your friend (or a sympathetic family member or friend) for help before you succumb.
- Don't eat in front of the television or computer, at the cinema, or in any other place where it's easy for hand-to-mouth movements to go on automatic pilot. (The exception to this rule is if you're having a single portion-controlled Atkins meal or bar.)

- Have substitute foods on hand. If a chocolate chip cookie can send you off the deep end, an Atkins Advantage bar should tame your chocolate lust.

FREQUENTLY ASKED QUESTIONS

Q. How do I get back on track after an "indiscretion"?
A. First of all, don't beat yourself up. We all have moments of weakness, and maybe that plate of chips your friend was eating was more than you could resist. Second, don't play the game of "Well, since I've already messed up, I might as well go the whole hog". For the rest of the day eat appropriately. Don't wait until tomorrow to get back on the wagon.

Q. What's carb creep?
A. Without realising it, as you gradually add foods, you may be consuming far more carbs than you think you are. This can make you complacent about your intake until your weight loss stalls. Once again, tracking your carbs and portion sizes should help you avoid carb creep.

Q. Why have my cravings returned?
A. Usually cravings vanish by the end of the first week on Induction when you convert to burning primarily fat for energy. There are several reasons why they may return. Women sometimes experience cravings a few days before their menstrual period. Going too long between meals, or adding foods such as dairy products or peanuts, may stimulate cravings. Stress can also destabilise blood sugar, triggering cravings for comfort foods. Adding a bit more fat, in the form of olives, half an avocado, or some cream cheese in a celery stick, can help you feel more satisfied, minimising cravings.

Q. Do I have to reintroduce all Phase 2 acceptable foods?
A. Of course not. If you don't like yoghurt or chickpeas or tomato juice, so be it. Or if a whole rung on the Carb Ladder holds no appeal for you, just skip it. There's still plenty of variety inherent in the wholefoods you can eat on Atkins.

Q. Why is my weight loss erratic?

A. As I've discussed with regard to plateaux, your body has its own schedule and won't share it with anyone. The important thing is to follow the programme faithfully and the pounds will come off. Again, adding exercise helps some people lose weight, but not everyone. Be sure to take your measurements weekly. If you've lost girth, the scales are bound to catch up.

Q. Why have I regained some of the weight I lost?

A. The reason I recommend that you not weigh yourself daily is that your weight can vary by as much as 2.2 kg (5 lb) even within a day. As long as you're following the programme, you should see some weight loss every week or so, unless you're on a plateau. If you stayed on track but gained a bit of weight since the previous week, you're probably retaining water or are constipated.

WHEN TO SAY GOODBYE TO PHASE 2

There are two big questions you'll face in the Balancing phase. The first we've alluded to throughout this chapter: "How do I find my personal carb balance, my threshold for consuming carbs while losing weight?" The answer? By trial and error! You'll gradually increase your daily Net Carb count. If weight loss levels off, you'll cut back by 5 grams of Net Carbs to see if it gets going again. When it does, you'll add another 5 grams, and so forth. You'll want to go as high as you can as long as weight loss continues, albeit more slowly than before, and you continue to feel good and in control of cravings. There is no right number, only the one that feels right for you and which you can maintain without too much effort.

The second, and related, question is, "When should I move to Phase 3?" If you've lost weight steadily and are now only about 4.5 kg (10 lb) from your goal weight, the answer is simple: now! Why? Because your long-term goal is to find a sustainable way of eating. And with 4.5 kg (10 lb) to go, you have enough time to try to reintroduce the remaining carb foods. If you aren't yet 4.5 kg (10 lb) from your goal, the answer is that it depends, just like when you were deciding when to move to Phase 2.

In that case, ask yourself which of these three scenarios describes you:

1. You've reached a daily intake of about 50 grams of Net Carbs, have introduced Phase 2 foods, and continue to slim down without experiencing cravings and unreasonable hunger. If so, feel free to move to Phase 3 now if you're eager for more variety in your meals. If you stall there, you can always return to Phase 2 to reboot weight loss.
2. You still have more than 4.5 kg (10 lb) to shed and are stalled in your weight-loss progress and/or experiencing cravings and extreme hunger before meals. By all means, stay in this phase until the cravings and hunger have vanished.
3. Although you lost weight in Phase 1, your progress in this phase has been frustrating, and some Phase 2 foods are creating cravings and undue hunger. You may have even gained a bit of weight. You may be extraordinarily sensitive to carbs and may have reached your carb tolerance at 30 or 35 grams of Net Carbs. Follow the advice above, be patient, and ramp up your activity level if possible.

Now let's meet Troy G., whose life seemed to be falling apart 11 years ago as he faced his excess weight, a serious gastrointestinal problem, and bankruptcy. Today, he's a lean ultra-marathon runner who knows that carb loading is not the only way to run a race. Read his story to get inspired to add fitness to your weight-loss programme.

In the next chapter, we'll move on to Phase 3, Pre-Maintenance, where you'll achieve your goal weight and begin the dress rehearsal for a lifetime of slimness.

ON THE RIGHT TRACK FOR GOOD

VITAL STATS

Daily Net Carb intake:
   60–70 grams
Age: 50
Height: 180 cm (5 ft 11 in)

Before weight: 104 kg
   (16 st 6 lb)
After weight: 73 kg
   (11 st 6 lb)
Weight lost: 31 kg (70 lb)

Troy G.'s life was in free fall. At the age of 39, he was an over-weight couch potato confronting his own health issues, and concerned about his wife, who had become partially disabled. Troy had lost his job and some business deals had gone wrong. The couple declared bankruptcy and their home was about to be repossessed. In the midst of these troubles, Troy started

Atkins, shed his excess weight within six months, and started running. Before long, his health was restored and he could boast a BMI of about 21. A new job took the family to College Station, Texas. Eleven years later, Troy remains committed to the Atkins lifestyle. Let's hear how he turned his life around.

I was always a skinny kid. When I played baseball in high school, I worked out and took supplements to bulk up. But in college I started living on pizza and beer, and after graduation I continued to live on junk food and my job as a software developer and programmer was a sedentary one. That skinny kid had become a heavy man. With everything out of control, I decided that the only things that I could control were my weight and my health.

I had lost weight before. After surgery to deal with diverticulitis, I was put on a liquid diet. I lost weight, but of course I regained it when I went back to eating solid food. One day when I was at my heaviest, I was playing peewee tackle football with my younger son, who was about 6 at the time.

I caught a pass and all I had to do was run a few metres to make the touchdown. Instead, I fell down. My son said, "Dad, would you play on the other team now?" That was my inspiration to be a role model for him by showing that you shouldn't give up on your goals.

I'd done what I thought was Atkins a couple of times before, but I was just cutting carbs without knowing what I was doing. This time I read *The New Atkins for a New You*, and my wife and I did Atkins together. We started with Induction and followed it to the letter. Although I've never been much for vegetables, I ate as much as I could, but can't say that I ever developed a taste for broccoli! I lost a pound and sometimes even two each day and never hit a plateau.

After three or four months I'd found how many carbs I could consume and keep losing weight, and within six months I was down 31 kg (70 lb). I was feeling so much better and more energetic that I decided to take up running. After a few months I began to enter 5-km (3-mile) races and then worked up to half marathons and finally marathons. This was all within a year of starting Atkins. Now I'm proud to call myself an ultra-marathon runner, having completed 21 marathons, as well as a dozen ultra-marathons (50 km/31 miles or greater). I've even run 113 km (70 miles) in a 24-hour period to match my weight loss of 31 kg (70 lb).

For many years I followed my low-carb lifestyle, but I was taking the conventional path of carb-loading before a race. I did okay, but I was always hitting the wall. After a marathon, I would feel like I had the ultimate hangover, but I continued to train that way. Then I did some research on how dietary fat provides more sustained energy than carbs and found that I could run on a low-carb regime. I'd been training that way for a couple of months and decided to try it on a 113 km (70-mile) celebratory run. I was able to do it by drinking Atkins shakes and taking breaks to rest or walk.

I was still not totally convinced that fat-loading was the way to go, but in the next marathon I tried it, and it was the easiest one I'd ever run. I usually hit the wall at the 32-km (20-mile) point, but this time I was able to actually run faster after that point than during the earlier part of the race.

My lucky number is now 70. It's my proof that you can take control of your life, that you can feel good about yourself and endure anything that is thrown at you. And 70 is also my personal proof that the Atkins lifestyle does work, not only for losing weight, but also for successfully preparing for endurance events.

I have to say that I've developed a totally different outlook on life. At 40 years old, I finally learned to distinguish between what I could control and focus on that, and to let go of what I couldn't control. The Atkins lifestyle helped me gain control of my life. And with regards to football, when my kids began their next peewee tackle season after I'd lost the 31.5 kg (70 lb), the coach didn't recognise me. And no one was suggesting I play for the other team!

Note: Troy has written a Nook eBook, *Endurance 70*, dedicated to the late Dr Atkins, about his experience as an endurance athlete. It is available at bn.com.

CHAPTER 7

THE FINISH LINE IS IN SIGHT

You're probably now just 4.5 kg (10 lb) from your goal weight, which you'll achieve in Phase 3, Pre-Maintenance (Fine-Tuning). Bravo! You've worked hard, been patient, and deserve the reward you're closing in on: a slim, healthy new you. I won't say the end is near, because reaching your goal weight is actually just the beginning of your new lifestyle. And if you've opted to begin this phase with more than 4.5 kg (10 lb) to go, you can still begin to broaden your food choices, although it may take you a bit longer to reach your goal weight.

TIME TO FINE-TUNE

When you moved to Phase 2 (Balancing), the trick was to go as slow as molasses (yes, I know it's an added sugar) – that is, gradually and deliberately. You'll do the same again as you see how much you can raise your daily Net Carb intake while exploring the final three rungs of the Carb Ladder (see page 14) in Phase 3 (Fine-Tuning). They include foods with the highest carb counts: fruits other than berries, cherries, and melon; starchy vegetables; and wholegrains, building on the foods lower on the Carb Ladder that you've already been eating. You might be able to eat all these "new" foods; another possibility, however, is that your metabolism may be able to handle only some of them – or small amounts. Or you may find that you can eat them rarely or not at all.

In this phase you'll come to understand how your body reacts to these foods in terms of slowing weight loss, halting it altogether, or prompting cravings or unreasonable hunger. All this is part of continuing to explore your tolerance for carbs while continuing to *lose* weight (what we call your personal carb balance) and then ultimately finding your slightly higher tolerance for carbs as you *maintain* weight loss.

PHASE 3 GUIDELINES

As you've already learned, the last thing you want to do is rush to add all the Phase 3 foods that you've been missing. After all, fruit, bread, potatoes, cereals, and grains are probably among the culprits that got you into trouble in the first place. Add them all at once and you'll almost certainly stall your fat-burning engine. But that's no reason to hang out in Phase 2. To stay in control, inch forwards until you discover how far you can go, and you'll know exactly what you can and cannot eat. Then make it your permanent way of eating to eliminate the struggles with weight you've experienced in the past. Much of the advice on how to succeed in Phase 3 will sound familiar, because it's the natural extension of Phase 2.

- Continue to consume a minimum of 12–15 grams of Net Carbs in the form of foundation vegetables, avoid foods with added sugar, have eight glasses of water or other acceptable fluids each day, and go no longer than three or four waking hours without eating, spreading out your carb intake across meals and snacks.
- Reintroduce new food groups one by one, following the Carb Ladder. Depending on your metabolism and weight-loss goal, this may be at weekly, fortnightly, or even longer intervals.
- Add carbohydrate foods within each rung of the Carb Ladder one by one. For example, reintroduce apples but gauge their impact, if any, for a couple of days before adding oranges.
- Increase your overall Net Carb intake in 10-gram increments (if you've been losing weight relatively easily) or 5-gram increments (if weight loss has slowed). Make these increases no more frequently than once a week; you can also do so every two weeks, or even less frequently.
- Continue to log your daily Net Carb intake in your journal, also noting any "new" foods so that you can ascertain if any of them are stalling your progress.
- Once you reach your goal weight, remain at that level of Net Carb intake for one month to ensure you can maintain it.
- Continue to weigh and measure yourself weekly.

Now let's review the acceptable Phase 3 foods, understanding that you may not be able to reintroduce all of them.

ACCEPTABLE PHASE 3 FOODS

OTHER FRUITS

Although legumes are acceptable in OWL, you may not have added them back yet. If so, do that before moving to fruit. (See pages 91–2 for suggestions.) On the other hand, if you're not big on lentils and other beans, simply skip them. As with the earlier lists of acceptable foods, the following include just a few representative foods on each rung of the Carb Ladder. Refer to the Atkins Carb Counter for more complete lists with serving sizes and Net Carb counts. Use the printed version available from Atkins, download it from atkins.com, or use the Atkins mobile app.

As with the berries, cherries, and melon that you reintroduced in OWL, have these higher-carb fruits in small quantities, starting with one at a time and only once a day. Have fresh or frozen (unsweetened) fruit or tinned fruit in water or juice rather than syrup. Avoid fruit juice and sweetened applesauce. Tropical fruits such as banana, mango, and plantain are considerably higher in carbs than other fruits, so wait on them until you see how you tolerate other fruits. As long as they're made without added sugar, small portions of jelly, jam, preserves, and fruit preserves made from Phase 3 fruits are also acceptable. (See "Low-Carb Resources" on page 184 for sources.)

- Apples
- Apricots
- Grapes
- Grapefruit
- Kiwi fruit
- Oranges
- Papayas
- Peaches or nectarines
- Pears
- Plums
- Pomegranates
- Watermelon

MAKE IT EASY

Save time by picking up packaged cut-up fresh fruit in the fruit and vegetables section. Divide the contents into appropriate portions to eat at home or take to work.

THE SCOOP ON SUGAR: FRESH VERSUS DRIED FRUIT

The process of drying fruit evaporates the water and concentrates the sugar content. Therefore, the amount of fresh fruit considered a single serving is not the same as a single serving of dried fruit. Compare the carb counts in the table below – dried fruits are shown in italics – and you'll see why they should be consumed in moderation.

FRUIT CARBS	AMOUNT AND TYPE	GRAMS OF NET
Apple	½ fresh	7.9
Apple	*30 g (1 oz) freeze-dried*	*23*
Banana	1 small fresh	20.4
Banana	*30 g (1 oz) freeze-dried*	*23*
Currants	50 g (2 oz) fresh	5.3
Currants	*2 tablespoons dried*	12.1
Grapes, Concord	50 g (2 oz)	7.5
Raisins	*1 tablespoon*	6.8
Mango	85 g (3 oz) fresh	11.1
Mango	*1 piece, freeze-dried*	*21*
Papaya	85 g (3 oz) fresh	6.6
Papaya	*1 strip, dried*	*12.2*

GO EASY ON FRUIT

Reintroduce fruit slowly and in small amounts, particularly if you've been craving it until now. To stay in control:

- Swap one serving of berries or melon for a serving of higher-carb fruits.
- Have no more than two fruit servings (including berries) a day.
- Always accompany fruit with some fat or protein.
- Start with the lower-carb fruits in this category, such as papayas, peaches, plums, or tangerines.
- Go "halfsies" by sharing an apple, pear, grapefruit, or papaya with a family member, or save the other half for tomorrow.

- Garnish your breakfast eggs with 50 g (2 oz) grapes or orange sections, or add them to a salad.
- Eat fruits such as bananas, pears, papayas, and mangos before they're very ripe, to minimise the impact on blood sugar.
- Combine higher-carb fruits in a fruit salad with lower-carb berries and/or melon.

STARCHY VEGETABLES

You've been eating plenty of foundation vegetables in the first two phases of the New Atkins Diet. After reintroducing other fruits, it's time to try to reintroduce the rest of the vegetable family. Like foundation vegetables, these roots, tubers, and other vegetables are high in fibre and antioxidants; however, they're higher in carbs. 110 g (4 oz) of baked acorn squash, for example, tallies 7.8 grams of Net Carbs; half a sweet potato and half a baked white potato contain 12.1 and 10.5 grams, respectively. Comparable servings of some tropical vegetables such as cassava (yuca), taro, and yautia are significantly higher in carbs.

Among the choices are:

- Beetroot
- Carrots
- Corn on (or off) the cob
- Jerusalem artichokes
- Peas
- Parsnips
- Potatoes, sweet and white
- Turnips
- Winter squash
- Yams

CURB THOSE CARBS

To enjoy some new vegetables without going overboard, try these ideas on for size:

- Have carrots raw instead of cooked, as cooking raises the carb count.
- Add 30 g (1 oz) grated carrot to tuna or chicken salad.
- Add grated carrots to cabbage slaw.
- Steam potatoes and cauliflower and mash together to mute the carb impact of potatoes.
- Make succotash with equal portions of frozen corn and edamame (instead of higher-carb butter beans).
- Roast a single cut-up potato or sweet potato with several foundation vegetables.
- Instead of squash soup, combine one part squash with twice as much pumpkin, which is actually a foundation veggie.
- Sauté 40 g (1½ oz) peas with sliced spring onions and thinly sliced lettuce.

WHOLEGRAINS

Occupying the top rung of the Carb Ladder, grains are the last wholefood group to be reintroduced. Not everyone can tolerate grains and products made with them, so proceed with caution. And don't confuse refined grains such as white flour and white rice with wholegrains. Baked goods, including bread, pitta, tortillas, biscuits, and cereals made with refined grains remain on the "avoid" list indefinitely (with the exception of low-carb products). Such products made with wholegrains are acceptable, but the Net Carb counts may vary greatly from one product to another. Here are some of the more common wholegrains:

- Barley
- Cornmeal
- Couscous, wholewheat
- Kasha (buckwheat groats)
- Wholemeal flour, wheat berries, bulgur, and cracked wheat
- Millet
- Oat bran and porridge oats (not instant)
- Quinoa
- Rice, brown, red, or wild

In Phase 3 you can also increase your daily intake of whole milk to 125 ml (4 fl oz), but continue to steer clear of low-fat milk and other low-fat dairy products. You can also experiment with low-carb products that have up to 9 grams of Net Carbs per serving. For an extended list of foods in these three rungs of the Carb Ladder, along with serving sizes and Net Carb gram counts, see the Atkins Carb Counter.

A LITTLE GOES A LONG WAY

When adding grains back into your diet, the best approach is to use very small portions, treating them as a garnish or a small component of a dish, rather than the star attraction. Instead of a conventional serving of a grain:

- Top a green salad with a little cooked wild rice, wheat berries, or other wholegrain.
- Combine equal proportions of cooked porridge oats, oat bran, and chopped nuts for a relatively low-carb hot breakfast.
- Swap the proportions of a grain salad by using a small amount of bulgur, quinoa, or kasha and plenty of chopped parsley, mint, spring onions, cucumber, and tomatoes.
- Mix a little cooked brown or wild rice into a stir-fry with courgettes, red peppers, and leftover chicken or beef.

FIND YOUR OWN PACE IN PHASE 3

As in the second phase, how individuals navigate the increase in food choices and grams of Net Carbs varies greatly. If you're still losing reliably each week, you may be able to move up in 10-gram increments and reintroduce all the food groups, one after another. Or you may need to use 5-gram increments some weeks and hang back at other times. If your tolerance for carbs is low and your weight loss has proceeded slowly or in fits and starts, it may take you considerably longer to introduce new foods. Someone with a high metabolism might have reached his or her goal weight and been able to reintroduce all rungs of the Carb Ladder after a month in Phase 3. Someone with a slow metabolism, in contrast, might take three months or more to get there and never reach the top of the Carb Ladder. Don't move to a higher carb count or add a new food group if you stop losing. Again, not everyone will be able to reintroduce all Phase 3 foods, or it could take several months to do so without stalling weight loss or provoking cravings and undue hunger.

WEEK-AT-A-GLANCE MEAL PLANS FOR PHASE 3

The following three plans continue to build progressively on one of the original meal plans, making it easy to reintroduce foods from the final three rungs of the Carb Ladder (see page 14). If you have reached these Net Carb daily levels but not reintroduced all the rungs of the Carb Ladder, your carb intake may differ from these sample meal plans. However, the three plans do illustrate how to gradually and progressively modify your intake as you climb the Carb Ladder and approach your goal weight.

WEEK-AT-A-GLANCE MEAL PLAN AT
50 GRAMS OF NET CARBS A DAY (Pages 138–139)

Continuing to evolve from the original Phase 1 meal plan, this plan assumes you've already reintroduced nuts and seeds, berries and other low-carb fruits, more dairy products, legumes, and tomato juice. It adds other fruits, swapping one serving of berries for higher-carb fruit, one at a time. As before, substitutions and additions are small and incremental, to make the transition as simple as possible. Easy suggestions for how to add these foods are indicated in **_boldface italic_** type in the meal plan on pages 138–139. Substitute other fruits for the items listed, if you prefer, using the Atkins Carb Counter to stay within the Net Carb guidelines.

WEEK AT-A-GLANCE MEAL PLAN AT 60 GRAMS OF NET CARBS A DAY (Pages 140–141)

The next rung on the Carb Ladder is reflected in the next evolution of the meal plan shown on pages 140–141, with a starchy vegetable sometimes taking the place of a foundation vegetable. Simple suggestions for how to add them appear in **_boldface italic_** type on the plan. Substitute other starchy vegetables with a comparable Net Carb count for those listed if you prefer, referring to the Atkins Carb Counter. However, remember that not everyone will be able to include starchy vegetables or this level of carb intake.

WEEK-AT-A-GLANCE MEAL PLAN AT 70 GRAMS OF NET CARBS A DAY (Pages 142–143)

The last meal plan (on pages 142–143) reintroduces wholegrains, the final rung of the Carb Ladder, building on the earlier plans. Simple suggestions for how to add these foods are indicated in **_boldface italic_** type in the meal plan. Not all people will be able to include wholegrains or this level of carb intake. If you find that you can go higher than 70 daily grams of Net Carbs, adjust the meal plan accordingly.

QUICK SNACKS FOR PHASE 3 AND BEYOND

Your snack options expand in Pre-Maintenance (Fine-Tuning), although you can continue to enjoy tasty, convenient Atkins snacks and shakes. If you have the ingredients in the fridge and store cupboard, you can also put together these tasty and portable snacks in minutes.

- Cottage cheese and orange slices
- Apple slices spread with almond or peanut butter
- Half a pear with blue cheese
- Greek yoghurt with papaya slices
- Atkins Trail Mix: nuts, seeds, no-sugar-added shredded coconut, and a cut-up Atkins bar
- Prosciutto-wrapped pineapple
- Provolone-wrapped kiwi slices
- Carrot sticks with hummus
- Air-popped popcorn sprinkled with grated Parmesan cheese.

EXERCISE: NO MORE EXCUSES

Okay, here I go again. Now that you're homing in on your goal weight, there's really no excuse not to add physical activity to your weight-control programme. It might speed the loss of those last few pounds, and without question it will help you maintain your soon-to-be-achieved new weight. If you've started exercising regularly, you're already on the right track. And if you've been working out all along, it might be time to intensify your efforts.

The NHS Live Well programme recommends that adults get a minimum of two and a half hours of moderate-intensity exercise a week. But any physical activity is better than none, and if you're new to exercise, you can certainly begin with less and gradually increase in intensity and duration. Make sure to include both resistance exercise, also known as strength training, to increase your muscle endurance and strength, and cardiovascular exercise. You can achieve the former with hand weights or resistance bands, or simply by using your body weight, as you do with push-ups. Brisk walking, jogging, swimming, and cycling are all great ways to achieve cardiovascular or aerobic exercise. Numerous websites offer videos and guided instruction.

Atkins Phase 3 (Fine-Tuning) Meal Plan at 50 g NC/day

	MONDAY	TUESDAY	WEDNESDAY	THURSDAY
BREAKFAST	2 eggs 40 g chopped onion 1 tsp olive oil 30 g Cheddar cheese *110 ml tomato juice* Net Carbs: 8.5 g; FV: 7.5 g	Atkins Advantage Chocolate Hazelnut Crunch Bar 25 almonds 5 large strawberries Net Carbs: 10.9 g; FV: 0 g	2 eggs 60–115 g ham 3 tbsp chopped onion 1 small tomato 50 g cantaloupe cubes *115 g Greek yoghurt* Net Carbs: 14.2 g; FV: 4.8 g	115 g steak or beef burger 1 tsp olive oil 90 g chopped pepper 40 g chopped onion 30 g Cheddar cheese 1 small tomato Net Carbs: 8.1 g; FV: 7.8 g
SNACK	Atkins Day Break Almond Cranberry Bar 10 almonds 5 large strawberries Net Carbs: 10.1 g; FV: 0 g	1 small tomato 30 g Cheddar cheese Net Carbs: 2.6 g; FV: 2.5 g	Atkins Day Break Cappuccino Nut Bar 10 walnut halves Net Carbs: 4.9 g; FV: 0 g	2 celery sticks 30 g Cheddar cheese Net Carbs: 2.2 g; FV: 2 g
LUNCH	115–175 g ham or pork chop 1 small tomato 30 g baby spinach 2 tbsp Vinaigrette* *½ medium pear* Net Carbs: 15.3 g; FV: 4 g	115–175 g chicken 1 small tomato 55 g mixed lettuce ½ avocado 2 tbsp Ranch Dressing* *40 g cooked chickpeas* Net Carbs: 13.9 g; FV: 5.1 g	115–175 g steak or beefburger 110 g mixed lettuce ½ avocado 2 tbsp Vinaigrette* *½ medium pear* Net Carbs: 15.3 g; FV: 4 g	Atkins Advantage Chocolate Decadence Bar 15 walnut halves *½ medium apple* Net Carbs: 12.6 g; FV: 0 g
SNACK	Atkins Advantage Café Royal RTD 10 almonds Net Carbs: 2.4 g; FV: 0 g	*½ medium pear* *110 g cottage cheese* Net Carbs: 15.1 g; FV: 0 g	1 small tomato 15 almonds *60 g hummus* Net Carbs: 9.1 g; FV: 2.5 g	25 almonds 80 g cantaloupe cubes *115 g Greek yoghurt* Net Carbs: 13.4 g; 0 g
DINNER	115–175 g tinned tuna or fish fillet 110 g mixed lettuce ½ avocado 2 tbsp Vinaigrette* 90 g broccoli 60 g chickpeas Net Carbs: 14.1 g; FV: 5.6 g	115–175 g steak or beef burger ½ medium pepper ⅓ small onion 55 g mixed lettuce 2 tbsp Ranch Dressing* Net Carbs: 6.3 g; FV: 5.5 g	115–175 g chicken 90 g broccoli florets 110 g mixed lettuce 2 tbsp Creamy Italian Dressing* Net Carbs: 4.5 g; FV: 4.3 g	115–175 g chicken 60 g baby spinach 45 g sliced pepper 1 small tomato 2 tbsp Ranch Dressing* 80 g cantaloupe cubes *25 g cooked lentils* Net Carbs: 14.5 g; FV: 5.8 g
	Total Net Carbs: 50.4 g Total Net Carbs from FV: 12.7 g	Total Net Carbs: 48.8 g Total Net Carbs from FV: 13.1 g	Total Net Carbs: 48 g Total Net Carbs from FV: 15.6 g	Total Net Carbs: 50.8 g Total Net Carbs from FV: 15.6 g

FRIDAY	SATURDAY	SUNDAY
30 g baby spinach	2 eggs	2 eggs
1 tsp olive oil	1 small tomato	60 g baby spinach
1 small tomato	60 g raspberries	1 tsp olive oil
½ avocado	*115 g Greek yoghurt*	½ pepper
30 g Cheddar cheese		30 g Cheddar cheese
		80 g cantaloupe cubes
Net Carbs: 5.3 g; FV: 5.3 g	Net Carbs: 12.5 g; FV: 2.5 g	Net Carbs: 12 g; FV: 5.3 g
Atkins Day Break Strawberry Yoghurt RTD	Atkins Day Break Strawberry Crisp Bar	1 celery stick
½ medium apple	15 almonds	30 g Cheddar cheese
	½ medium pear	*110 ml tomato juice*
Net Carbs: 11.5 g; FV: 0 g	Net Carbs: 15.7 g; FV: 0 g	Net Carbs: 5.7 g; FV: 5.4 g
115–175 g chicken	115–175 g tinned tuna or fish fillet	Atkins Advantage Dark Chocolate Crunch Bar
110 g mixed greens	2 tbsp mayonnaise or tartar sauce	20 walnut halves
45 g sliced pepper	1 celery stick	*½ medium apple*
2 tbsp Creamy Italian Dressing*	40 g chopped pepper	
40 g cooked chickpeas	1 small tomato	
	15 walnut halves	
Net Carbs: 15.6 g; FV: 4.5 g	Net Carbs: 7.1 g; FV: 5 g	Net Carbs: 15 g; FV: 0 g
Atkins Advantage Milk Chocolate RTD	2 celery sticks	90 g chopped pepper
15 almonds	2 tbsp Creamy Italian Dressing*	1 tbsp Ranch Dressing*
		25 almonds
Net Carbs: 3 g; FV: 0 g	Net Carbs: 2.2 g; FV: 2 g	Net Carbs: 5.4 g; FV: 2.2 g
115–175 g ham or pork chop	115–175 g steak or beef burger	175 g chicken
90 g broccoli	30 g Cheddar cheese	90 g broccoli
55 g mixed lettuce	1 small tomato	1 tsp olive oil
2 tbsp Creamy Italian Dressing*	½ avocado	55 g mixed lettuce
10 walnut halves	½ small onion	½ avocado
110 g cottage cheese	*25 g cooked lentils*	2 tbsp Vinaigrette*
5 large strawberries		*60 g chickpeas*
Net Carbs: 13.8 g; FV: 5.8 g	Net Carbs: 14.4 g; FV: 6.5 g	Net Carbs: 12.7 g; FV: 4.2 g
Total Net Carbs: 49.2 g	Total Net Carbs: 51.9 g	Total Net Carbs: 50.8 g
Total Net Carbs from FV: 15.6 g	Total Net Carbs from FV: 16 g	Total Net Carbs from FV: 17.1 g

Atkins Phase 3 (Fine-Tuning) Meal Plan at 60 g NC/day

	MONDAY	TUESDAY	WEDNESDAY	THURSDAY
BREAKFAST	2 eggs 40 g chopped onion 1 tsp olive oil 30 g Cheddar cheese 110 ml tomato juice	Atkins Advantage Chocolate Hazelnut Crunch Bar 25 almonds 7 large strawberries	2 eggs 3 tbsp chopped onion 1 small tomato 50 g cantaloupe cubes 115 g Greek yoghurt	115–175 g steak or beef burger 1 tsp olive oil 90 g chopped pepper 40 g chopped onion 30 g Cheddar cheese 110 ml tomato juice
	Net Carbs: 8.5 g; FV: 7.5 g	Net Carbs: 10.9 g; FV: 0 g	Net Carbs: 14.1 g; FV: 4.8 g	Net Carbs: 10 g; FV: 9.7 g
SNACK	Atkins Day Break Almond Cranberry Bar 10 almonds 5 large strawberries	1 small tomato 30 g Cheddar cheese	Atkins Day Break Cappuccino Nut Bar 10 walnut halves	1 medium carrot 60 g hummus
	Net Carbs: 10.1 g; FV: 0 g	Net Carbs: 2.6 g; FV: 2.5 g	Net Carbs: 4.9 g; FV: 0 g	Net Carbs: 9.1 g; FV: 0 g
LUNCH	115–175 g ham or pork chop 1 small tomato 30 g baby spinach 2 tbsp Vinaigrette* *80 g peas*	115–175 g chicken 1 small tomato 55 g mixed lettuce ½ avocado 2 tbsp Ranch Dressing* 40 g cooked chickpeas	115–175 g steak or beefburger 110 g mixed lettuce ½ avocado 2 tbsp Vinaigrette* ½ medium pear	Atkins Advantage Chocolate Decadence Bar 15 walnut halves ½ medium apple
	Net Carbs: 11.3 g; FV: 4 g	Net Carbs: 13.9 g; FV: 5.1 g	Net Carbs: 15.3 g; FV: 4 g	Net Carbs: 12.6 g; FV: 0 g
SNACK	Atkins Advantage Café Royal RTD 10 almonds ½ medium pear	½ medium apple 110 g cottage cheese	1 small tomato 15 almonds 60 g hummus	25 almonds 80 g cantaloupe cubes 115 g Greek yoghurt
	Net carbs: 13.4 g; FV: 0 g	Net Carbs: 15.1 g; FV: 0 g	Net Carbs: 9.1 g; FV: 2.5 g	Net Carbs: 13.4 g; FV: 0 g
DINNER	115–175 g tinned tuna or fish fillet 110 g mixed lettuce ½ avocado 2 tbsp Vinaigrette* 90 g broccoli 55 g cooked chickpeas	115–175 g steak or beefburger ½ pepper ⅓ small onion 55 g mixed lettuce 2 tbsp Ranch Dressing* *80 g peas* 110 ml tomato juice	115–175 g chicken 90 g broccoli 110 g mixed lettuce 2 tbsp Creamy Italian Dressing* *80 g peas* *55 g cooked carrots*	115–175 g chicken 30 g baby spinach 45 g sliced pepper 1 small tomato 2 tbsp Ranch Dressing* 50 g cantaloupe cubes 25 g cooked lentils
	Net Carbs: 15.8 g; FV: 5.6 g	Net Carbs: 17.6 g; FV: 9.9 g	Net Carbs: 15.6 g; FV: 4.3 g	Net Carbs: 14.5 g; FV: 5.8 g
	Total Net Carbs: 59.1 g Total Net Carbs from FV: 17.1 g	Total Net Carbs: 60.1 g Total Net Carbs from FV: 17.5 g	Total Net Carbs: 59 g Total Net Carbs from FV: 15.6 g	Total Net Carbs: 59.6 g Total Net Carbs from FV: 15.5 g

FRIDAY	SATURDAY	SUNDAY
30 g baby spinach	2 eggs	2 eggs
1 tsp olive oil	1 small tomato	60 g baby spinach
1 small tomato	60 g raspberries	1 tsp olive oil
½ avocado	115 g Greek yoghurt	½ pepper
30 g Cheddar cheese		30 g Cheddar cheese
110 ml tomato juice		80 g cantaloupe cubes
Net Carbs: 9.7 g; FV: 9.7 g	Net Carbs: 12.5 g; FV: 2.5 g	Net Carbs: 12 g; FV: 5.3 g
Atkins Day Break Strawberry Yoghurt RTD	Atkins Day Break Strawberry Crisp Bar	2 celery sticks
½ medium apple	15 almonds	30 g Cheddar cheese
	½ medium pear	110 ml tomato juice
Net Carbs: 11.5 g; FV: 0 g	Net Carbs: 15.7 g; FV: 0 g	Net Carbs: 6.7 g; FV: 6.4 g
115–175 g chicken	115–175 g tinned tuna or fish fillet	Atkins Advantage Dark Chocolate Crunch Bar
110 g mixed lettuce	2 tbsp mayonnaise or tartare sauce	20 walnut halves
45 g sliced pepper	45 g chopped pepper	½ medium pear
2 tbsp creamy Italian dressing*	1 small tomato	
55 g cooked chickpeas	15 walnut halves	
Net Carbs: 15.6 g; FV: 4.5 g	Net Carbs: 6.1 g; FV: 4 g	Net Carbs: 15 g; FV: 0 g
Atkins Advantage Milk Chocolate RTD	1 medium carrot	90 g chopped pepper
15 almonds	2 tbsp creamy Italian dressing	60 g hummus
		25 almonds
Net Carbs: 3 g; FV: 0 g	Net Carbs: 4.4 g; FV: 0 g	Net Carbs: 10 g; FV: 2.2 g
115–175 g ham or pork chop	115 g steak or beef burger	175 g chicken
90 g broccoli	1 small tomato	90 g broccoli
110 g mixed lettuce	½ avocado	55 g mixed lettuce
25 g chickpeas	½ small onion, sliced	½ avocado
2 tbsp Creamy Italian Dressing*	½ baked sweet potato	2 tbsp Vinaigrette*
10 walnut halves	80 g peas	80 g peas
110 g cottage cheese		80 g cooked carrot
7 large strawberries		
25 g grated carrot		
Net Carbs: 21 g; FV: 4.3 g	Net Carbs: 21 g; FV: 6.5 g	Net Carbs: 15.7 g; FV: 4.2 g
Total Net Carbs: 60.7 g	Total Net Carbs: 59.7 g	Total Net Carbs: 59.4 g
Total Net Carbs from FV: 18.5 g	Total Net Carbs from FV: 13 g	Total Net Carbs from FV: 18.1 g

Atkins Phase 3 (Fine-Tuning) Meal Plan at 70 g NC/day

	MONDAY	TUESDAY	WEDNESDAY	THURSDAY

BREAKFAST	2 eggs
	40 g chopped onion
	1 tsp olive oil
	30 g Cheddar cheese
	110 ml tomato juice
	
	Net Carbs: 8.5 g; FV: 7.5 g
		Atkins Advantage Chocolate
		   Hazelnut Crunch Bar
		25 almonds
		7 large strawberries
		
		Net Carbs: 10.9 g; FV: 0 g
			2 eggs
			3 tbsp chopped onion
			1 small tomato
			50 g cantaloupe cubes
			115 g Greek yoghurt
			
			Net Carbs: 14.1 g; FV: 4.8 g
				115–175 g steak or beef
				   burger
				1 tsp olive oil
				90 g chopped pepper
				40 g chopped onion
				30 g Cheddar cheese
				110 ml tomato juice
				Net Carbs: 10 g; FV: 9.7 g

SNACK	Atkins Day Break Almond
	   Cranberry Bar
	10 almonds
	5 large strawberries
	Net Carbs: 10.1 g; FV: 0 g
		2 celery sticks
		30 g Cheddar cheese
		110 ml tomato juice
		
		Net Carbs: 6.5 g; FV: 6.4 g
			Atkins Day Break
			   Cappuccino Nut Bar
			10 walnut halves
			
			Net Carbs: 4.9 g; FV: 0 g
				1 medium carrot
				60 g hummus
				4 wholegrain crackers
				
				Net Carbs: 20 g; FV: 0 g

LUNCH	115–175 g ham or pork chop
	1 small tomato
	30 g baby spinach
	2 tbsp Vinaigrette*
	80 g peas
	50 g brown rice
	Net Carbs: 21.9 g; FV: 4 g
		115–175 g chicken
		1 small tomato
		55 g mixed lettuce
		½ avocado
		2 tbsp Ranch Dressing*
		40 g cooked chickpeas
		Net Carbs: 13.9 g; FV: 5.1 g
			115–175 g steak or
			   beefburger
			110 g mixed lettuce
			½ avocado
			2 tbsp Vinaigrette*
			½ medium pear
			Net Carbs: 15.3 g; FV: 4 g
				Atkins Advantage Chocolate
				   Decadence Bar
				15 almonds
				½ medium apple
				
				Net Carbs: 12.2 g; FV: 0 g

SNACK	Atkins Advantage Café Royal RTD 10 almonds ½ medium pear Net Carbs: 13.4 g; FV: 0 g	½ medium pear 110 g cottage cheese Net Carbs: 15.1 g; FV: 0 g	1 small tomato 60 g hummus *4 wholegrain crackers* Net Carbs: 18.3 g; FV: 2.5 g	25 almonds 80 g cantaloupe cubes 115 g Greek yoghurt Net Carbs: 13.4 g; FV: 0 g

DINNER	115–175 g tinned tuna or
	   fish fillet
	110 g mixed lettuce
	½ avocado
	2 tbsp Vinaigrette*
	90 g broccoli
	55 g cooked chickpeas
	Net carbs: 16.8 g; FV: 5.6 g
		115–175 g steak or beef
		   burger
		½ medium pepper
		⅓ small onion
		55 g mixed lettuce
		2 tbsp Ranch Dressing*
		80 g peas
		50 g brown rice
		Net Carbs: 23.9 g; FV: 5.5 g
			115–175 g chicken
			90 g broccoli
			110 g mixed lettuce
			2 tbsp Creamy Italian
			   Dressing*
			80 g peas
			55 g cooked sliced carrots
			Net Carbs: 15.6 g; FV: 4.3 g
				115–175 g chicken
				30 g baby spinach
				45 g pepper
				1 small tomato
				2 tbsp Ranch Dressing*
				80 g cantaloupe cubes
				25 g cooked lentils
				Net Carbs: 14.5 g; FV: 5.8 g

	Total Net Carbs: 70.7 g
	Total Net Carbs from FV:
	   17.1 g
		Total Net Carbs: 70.3 g
		Total Net Carbs from FV: 17 g
			Total Net Carbs: 68.2 g
			Total Net Carbs from FV:
			   15.6 g
				Total Net Carbs: 70.1 g
				Total Net Carbs from FV:
				   15.5 g

FRIDAY	SATURDAY	SUNDAY
60 g baby spinach	2 eggs	2 eggs
1 tsp olive oil	1 small tomato	60 g baby spinach
1 small tomato	60 g raspberries	1 tsp olive oil
½ avocado	115 g Greek yoghurt	½ red pepper
30 g Cheddar cheese		30 g Cheddar cheese
110 ml tomato juice		80 g cantaloupe cubes
Net Carbs: 11.1 g; FV: 11.2 g	Net Carbs: 12.5 g; FV: 2.5 g	Net Carbs: 12 g; FV: 5.3 g
Atkins Day Break Strawberry Yoghurt RTD	Atkins Day Break Strawberry Crisp Bar	30 g Cheddar cheese
½ medium pear	15 almonds	110 ml tomato juice
	½ medium pear	1 medium carrot
Net Carbs: 14 g; FV: 0 g	Net Carbs: 15.7 g; FV: 0 g	Net Carbs: 8.9 g; FV: 4.4 g
115–175 g chicken	115–175 g tinned tuna or fish fillet	Atkins Advantage Chocolate Crunch Bar
110 g mixed lettuce	2 tbsp mayonnaise or tartare sauce	10 walnut halves
65 g pepper	45 g chopped pepper	½ medium apple
2 tbsp Creamy Italian Dressing*	1 small tomato	
½ small baked potato	10 walnut halves	
	4 wholegrain crackers	
Net Carbs: 18.8 g; FV: 5.5 g	Net Carbs: 16.3 g; FV: 4 g	Net Carbs: 13.6 g; FV: 0 g
Atkins Advantage Milk Chocolate RTD	1 medium carrot	135 g chopped pepper
15 almonds	2 tbsp Creamy Italian Dressing*	60 g hummus
		25 almonds
Net Carbs: 3 g; FV: 0 g	Net Carbs: 4.4 g; FV: 0 g	Net Carbs: 10.6 g; FV: 2.8 g
115–175 g ham or pork chop	115–175 g steak or beef burger	175 g chicken
90 g broccoli	1 small tomato	90 g broccoli
110 g mixed lettuce	½ avocado	110 g mixed lettuce
55 g cooked chickpeas	½ small onion, sliced	½ avocado
2 tbsp Creamy Italian Dressing	½ baked sweet potato	2 tbsp Vinaigrette*
25 g grated carrot	**80 g peas**	80 g peas
25 almonds		80 g cooked carrots
		50g brown rice
Net Carbs: 21.9 g; FV: 4.3 g	Net Carbs: 21 g; FV: 6.5 g	Net Carbs: 23.5 g; FV: 5.6 g
Total Net Carbs: 68.8 g	Total Net Carbs: 69.9 g	Total Net Carbs: 68.6 g
Total Net Carbs from FV: 21 g	Total Net Carbs from FV: 13 g	Total Net Carbs from FV: 18.1 g

WHAT TO EXPECT

The closer you get to your goal weight, the more your body resists letting go of its excess baggage. Take the following into consideration:

- *You may want to adjust your goal.* If you feel good about yourself at the weight you've achieved, terrific. You may have reached your natural weight, which is the one you can maintain easily. Or perhaps your original goal was too modest and you've realised that you could actually shave off even more weight now that you've experienced such success on Atkins. If so, there's no reason not to dial your goal weight down another 4.5 kg (10 lb) or so.
- *Take a break.* Or you may decide to hang out at a certain weight for a few months, get comfortable with it, and then take off the final 4.5 kg (10 lb).
- *It's not just about weight.* Another possibility is that although your weight is a bit higher than you'd originally aimed for, you've lost inches and can fit into clothes you haven't worn in years. The point is that there is no magic number, just the right one for you.
- *You'll need to experiment to find your limits.* Figuring out which foods you can or cannot handle is important for long-term weight control. Wouldn't you rather know for a fact that eating potatoes or bananas just isn't worth the price?
- *Your weight loss may slow to a crawl.* This is both deliberate – so that you can expand your carb intake and food choices – and natural. Weight loss obviously slows the closer you get to where your body naturally "wants" to be. And losing slowly gives you time to get really comfortable as you move to a permanent way of eating.

TROUBLESHOOTING

Even though you're almost at your goal, adding carbs and new foods can cause some frustrations. Here's how to handle them – or accept them.

- *You may experience cravings and uncontrollable hunger* as you add foods you have not eaten in some time. See page 144 for how to proceed.

- *You may end up on a plateau.* If you've already experienced one or more plateaux in OWL, you know all about that exercise in delayed gratification. If you've been spared this frustrating experience to date, my advice is to first ascertain that it's truly a plateau, meaning you're doing everything correctly. If so, reduce your daily Net Carb intake by 10 grams and wait it out as patiently as you can.
- *You may stumble upon your Net Carb tolerance for weight maintenance* in what initially appears to be a plateau. To see if this is the case, step down 10 grams of Net Carbs daily for at least a week. If weight loss resumes, go up another 5 grams, and so forth.

MISSION ACCOMPLISHED? NOT QUITE

The day you've dreamed of for months has finally arrived. You've reached your goal weight! Whether you've melted away 9 kg (20 lb), shed 23 kg (50 lb), or joined the bye-bye-45 kg (100-lb) club, congratulations on a job well done. Can you sit back and relax? Sure. Can you pat yourself on the back? Absolutely. Can you celebrate by pigging out on all those foods you've forsaken for the duration? No way! In fact, you aren't even ready to leave Phase 3 yet. Why? As the old saying goes, losing weight is easy; the hard part is maintaining your new weight. That's exactly what you begin to do in Phase 3, and that's why this phase is considered a dress rehearsal for Phase 4, Lifetime Maintenance. For the next four weeks your job is to maintain your goal weight.

PRACTICE MAKES PERFECT

To stay at your new weight, you need to know exactly how many grams of Net Carbs you can eat each day. Hint: it's usually 5 or 10 grams higher than the highest personal carb balance number you achieved while still losing weight. You'll also be assessing the ease or difficulty of keeping your weight constant at that level. The highest level of carb intake you can push yourself to may not be the level at which you're most comfortable.

In addition to monitoring your weight for the next month, stay alert to those old familiar indicators that you know all too well from when you began Atkins: low energy, carb cravings, and unreasonable hunger. If you're dragging around, feeling jittery, lusting after certain foods, or ravenous by the time your next meal or snack rolls around, chances are you've pushed yourself too high. It's likely you're also having a hard time maintaining your new weight at this unsustainable level, although a swing of a kilo or a couple of pounds from day to day is normal. Continue to use weight averaging instead of a single day's weight as an indicator.

If you're struggling to maintain your weight at this level, simply back down by 5 grams of Net Carbs daily and see if that's easier to handle. If that doesn't do the job, go down another 5 grams. This process may involve some trial and error, during which you may also find that you've reintroduced certain foods that are giving you problems, perhaps by stimulating cravings or uncontrollable hunger. If you suspect that particular foods are sabotaging your progress, eliminate them for several days to see whether things improve before trying to introduce them again.

Once you find the number of grams of Net Carbs that's sustainable in terms of weight maintenance and the other indicators discussed above, remain at that level for four weeks before moving to Phase 4. Just to be clear, don't leave Phase 3 until your weight has remained constant for four weeks! This back-and-forth business may seem like a drag now that you've reached your goal weight. But knowing exactly what you can and cannot handle enables you to stay in control in the coming months – and years.

FREQUENTLY ASKED QUESTIONS

Q. How do I know when I've reached the right weight for me?
A. There is no single right or wrong weight. Your body type, age, hormonal status, activity level, and genetics all play a role. As we've discussed, you may be able to achieve a lower weight, but if it's a struggle to maintain it, you may want to accept that being 2.2 kg (5 lb) or even 4.5 kg (10 lb) heavier is where your body naturally wants to be. Again, girth counts as much as weight. As you tone your abdominals and other muscles with regular physical activity, your body will appear slimmer. When you come to a point where you're comfortable with your weight at this time in your life, that's the place to remain.

Q. Can I eat any low-carb product when I'm in Phase 3?
A. In Phase 1, you can have low-carb foods with Net Carb counts of 3 grams per serving; that increases to 6 grams per serving in OWL, and to 9 grams in this phase. In Lifetime Maintenance, the number rises to 10 grams or more, assuming your carb tolerance allows.

Q. Can I have more than one or two glasses of wine now that I have reached my goal weight?
A. Yes, if it doesn't cause weight gain or leave you vulnerable to overeating the snack foods that often accompany alcohol. I generally recommend a single glass for women and up to two for men, but you know your own tolerance. If you regain weight or lose control, drop back to a single glass or none. Also continue to avoid high-carb beer and mixers made with added sugar.

Q. Why am I experiencing cravings I haven't had for months?
A. There are two possible explanations. Either you're simply eating too many carbs and not burning primarily fat for energy anymore (remember, fat burning suppresses your appetite) or you've reintroduced a food or food group that's spiking your blood sugar. Fruit may be the culprit, particularly if you're not accompanying it with fat or protein to moderate the impact on your blood sugar. Cut back by 10 grams of Net Carbs a day and eliminate the foods you're added recently. Then reintroduce them slowly, one by one, to find out which ones are creating cravings.

Q. How can I tame my sweet tooth?
A. There are two approaches: satisfy it or eliminate it. Satisfy your sweet tooth with acceptable substitutes, such as an Atkins Endulge bar. If you're able to have such treats without overdoing them and without causing cravings, fine. If not, eliminate any foods that may be triggering cravings for sweets until you get the situation under control.

Q. What puddings can I have in this phase?
A. In addition to Endulge bars, plus the berries, cherries, and melon you started to eat in Phase 2, you can have almost any other fruit, as well as other puddings with no added sugar and no more than 9 grams of Net Carbs.

MOVING ON

The big question, of course, is how to know when to move to Phase 4, Lifetime Maintenance. If you can answer all the following questions in the affirmative, go ahead. Otherwise, hold off until you have three yeses.

- Are you at your goal or adjusted goal weight?
- Has your weight remained constant for the last four weeks?
- Are cravings and undue hunger no longer a problem?

Before you get to Chapter 8, where you'll learn how to transition from a weight-loss programme to a weight-maintenance programme – that means the rest of your slim, energised, healthy life! – meet Gretchen M. Her ongoing weight-loss journey on Atkins is nothing less than amazing.

She has already lost an unbelievable 136 kg (300 lb) and still has another 48 kg (100 lb) to go. When you read her story you'll be as convinced as I am that she'll reach her goal weight – and stay there! Gretchen knows for a fact that she will never fall back into her old life. "I've been through it all and nothing will make me go back to the bad old days," she declares.

HITTING BOTTOM BEFORE
SEEING THE LIGHT

VITAL STATS

Daily Net Carb intake: 25–35
   grams
Age: 37
Height: 185 cm (6ft 1 in)

Before weight: 255 kg
   (40 st 3 lb)
(estimated)
After weight: 118 kg
   (18 st 9 lb)
Lost: 137 kg (300 lb)

Gretchen M. of Las Vegas has had it tough, starting with a childhood shaped by an alcoholic father and an abusive mother. Her marriage was not much better. Serious health problems, the loss of her career, and having to send her children away all caused the emotional distress that contributed to her obesity. But then Gretchen found Atkins. She's lost a remarkable amount of weight and knows the rest is just a matter of time. She credits Atkins with helping her turn her life around. Gretchen shares her painful but ultimately transformative life story.

My doctor would never give me my starting weight because he thought it would demotivate me and no scale could hold me, so I'm not really sure how much I weighed at my heaviest. I needed instant gratification, so instead of setting a goal weight at the start I set mini goals, beginning with 2.2-kg (5-lb) losses; later, with every 4.5 kg (10 lb) I lost, I'd buy myself a charm for my weight-loss charm bracelet. I also took a picture of myself every three or four weeks in the same shirt after visiting my doctor and getting my current weight, and post both on my Facebook page.

Although I'm tall and I was always curvy, after I had my two children I could never get below 91 kg (200 lb). I was a nurse, but I crushed my knee and became addicted to painkillers, which ended that career. I then found a part-time job without benefits. Meanwhile, my husband and I divorced. Shortly afterward, I was diagnosed with cancer. The kids and I were living with my mother, but she couldn't handle the stress of my situation, so she kicked us out. Painful as this was, it was no surprise. When my father was dying of cancer years ago, my mother made me care for him. She beat me every day (and forbade me to cry) before I left home at 15.

I was unable to provide a decent place to live while I was undergoing chemo and radiation, so I signed over custody of my son and daughter to my ex's parents. They lived in Idaho, so I rarely saw the kids. One bright spot in this list of horrors was meeting my boyfriend six months before my cancer diagnosis. He has been by my side the whole time.

Over the Christmas holidays of 2010, I had my kids with me and we went shopping. I was so heavy I could barely walk and sweat was pouring off me. My son was taking forever to decide which shirt to get and mouthed off at me. I completely lost it and screamed at him. Everyone stared at us and I could tell by the look on both kids' faces that they were ashamed of me. It just tore me apart. After they left to go back to Idaho, I was this close to killing myself. Instead, I got up at five o'clock the next morning, went online, and found Atkins.

When I read about carbohydrates it was as though a lightbulb went on in my head. I've since changed my entire way of eating. Now if God made it, I eat it, meaning no sugar and no processed foods. When I eat out I know which questions to ask and what to order, but I prefer my own food because I know exactly what's in it.

I'm in Phase 2 now and my goal is to get to 72 kg (11 st 4 lb), which means losing another 48 kg (105 lb). I've already lost almost three times that, so I know I can do it. I'm very active, walking my dog like 12 times a day and working out regularly on a stationary bike.

I've survived an abusive childhood, a horrible marriage, destroying my knee, and losing my career, but now I know there's nothing I can't accomplish. Sometimes I have bad days, but now I can handle what once would have triggered a binge. As long as I follow Atkins, I can stay in control. I don't have to fill myself up to feel good. My brain is the calmest it has ever been. I don't understand it, but I live it!

I used to wear size 7X or 8X clothing (UK oversize 38–42), and even that was skintight on me. As I lost weight, I began to sell my fat-lady clothes on eBay. Then I branched out, finding other large-sized items, and now have a thriving e-business. This new career has opened up a whole new world for me. More important, my cancer is in remission, my 16-year-old daughter is back home, and my son's in college, heading for law school. And when I look at my kids all I see is pride, not embarrassment, in their eyes.

MAKE IT EASY

I cook one day a week and freeze meals so I always have something I can pop in the microwave. One of my favourite snacks is whole-milk yoghurt with peeled, sliced cucumbers. *-GM*

CHAPTER 8

WELCOME THE NEW YOU

You did it! You're finally in Phase 4, Lifetime Maintenance. You set a goal, made significant changes in your habits, stuck to your guns, and accomplished what you set out to do. You're probably receiving compliments left and right, along with looks of amazement from people who haven't seen you in a while. Exciting as all that attention can be, it's probably nothing compared with your own sense of pride and accomplishment. Pat yourself on the back and take a bow! And carve out time to celebrate your achievements, perhaps with some new form-fitting clothes, a weekend at the beach, or a great new haircut and makeover. I also strongly recommend that you record your feelings about your weight-loss journey and the happy results in your journal. And don't forget to take an "after" photo of the svelte new you! When you think about your accomplishments, don't stop with your streamlined body. If any of the following apply, congratulate yourself on them as well. For example, in the process of doing Atkins, did you do any of the following?

- Eliminate a destructive habit such as drinking sugary fizzy drinks, eating in front of the television, or having a daily doughnut at break time.
- Develop a healthy new habit of a daily brisk walk or riding your bike to work, or start an exercise programme or build upon an existing one.
- Create weekly meal plans and shopping lists.

- Develop a love of vegetables.
- Improve your family's nutrition and sit down together for meals more often.
- Honour your commitments to yourself.
- Make other significant and positive changes in your life.

THE LONG HAUL

In your current cloud of optimism you may be saying to yourself, "I've lost the weight and kept it off for a month, so what's the point of yet another phase of Atkins?" Whoa! That kind of thinking can set you up for a fall. Again, the last four weeks of Pre-Maintenance were only a rehearsal for Lifetime Maintenance, which is not so much a phase as a permanent lifestyle. Sad to say, this is where all too many people, regardless of how they lost weight, get cocky and soon find themselves in trouble. In fact, up to 95 per cent of people who shed extra weight on any weight-loss programme regain it when they return to their old eating habits. Or they fall off the wagon and can't figure out how to climb back on. According to the National Weight Control Registry in the US, people who keep off their lost pounds have several traits in common. They:

- Eat breakfast
- Exercise almost every day
- Monitor their weight regularly
- Track their food intake.

The good news is that if you're following the Atkins programme and you've opted to make physical fitness part of your life, there's no reason why you have to become part of that 95 per cent. In many additional ways, Atkins is designed to make maintaining your weight easy.

Here's why:

- You've moved from phase to phase, gradually increasing your carb intake, as you worked towards a permanent way of eating.
- By reintroducing foods one by one, you know which, if any, could spell trouble for you.

- You now know which foods you can do without and which you love but must eat in moderation.
- You've learned how to be alert to the signals of cravings or undue hunger and how to respond before you lose control.
- You've discovered how to substitute certain low-carb foods for high-carb ones, treat other foods as garnishes, and more.
- Most important, you've come to trust the Atkins programme and experience the pleasure of feeling good, both physically and emotionally.

If you accept that Phase 4 is a lifestyle and act accordingly, I can promise that you'll never have to "diet" again. Does that mean that you won't ever regain a bit of weight? Of course not. If you go on holiday and eat out every night, you may well pack on some excess baggage. If an injury lays you up for a few weeks and you can't get to your exercise class, some excess weight may creep back. But now you possess the tools and skills, the same ones you've honed for months, to turn around any such situation. Just as important, don't succumb to negative thinking by letting an occasional misstep become a reason to wallow in guilt and punish yourself by falling into a downwards spiral.

ACCEPTABLE PHASE 4 FOODS

In general, the foods you can eat in Lifetime Maintenance are the same ones you've already been eating. There may be some foods you tried to reintroduce earlier without success that you can now handle. Feel free to experiment at any time as long as your weight remains under control. Just as there's great variation in how many carbs people can consume while losing weight, the same applies to weight maintenance. You might not be able to get much beyond 50 or 55 grams of Net Carbs a day (or even less), or you might be humming along at close to 100 grams or more.

FOOLPROOF ADVICE ON WEIGHT MAINTENANCE

To remain in control of your hard-won new weight:

- Stay at your carb tolerance level, the number of daily grams of Net Carbs you can consume while maintaining your weight.

This is the threshold you discovered when you maintained your weight for a month in Phase 3 (Fine-Tuning).

- Continue to have a minimum of 12–15 grams of Net Carbs in the form of foundation vegetables.
- Continue to have 115–175 g (4–6 oz) of (cooked) protein at each meal.
- Aim for no more than two servings of fruit a day.
- Continue to see fat as your friend and integral to weight management.
- Combine carbohydrate foods with fat and/or protein to moderate your blood-sugar response.
- Continue to drink plenty of water and other non-caloric beverages.
- Adjust your carb intake if you become less (or more) active.
- Distinguish between hunger and habit.
- Continue to weigh and measure yourself once a week.
- Never let yourself gain more than 2.2 kg (5 lb) – unless you become pregnant – without taking immediate action.
- Add new foods one at a time to gauge their impact on cravings and appetite.
- Engage in regular physical activity.
- Portion out ahead of time any foods, such as nuts or cheese, that you might be tempted to overeat.
- Keep reading labels, especially on any new foods.
- Stay alert to the possibility of carb creep.
- Plan ahead if you decide to take an occasional departure from your low-carb lifestyle. (See "Taking a Break", pages 159–160.)

APPETITE ADJUSTMENT

Now that you're maintaining rather than losing weight, you'll be consuming a slightly larger (with the emphasis on slightly) quantity of food, meaning more daily calories. Your appetite will also increase slightly at this point. As long as you're close to the weight your body "wants" to be, this is likely to occur naturally. Does that mean you'll also be consuming more carbs than you were in the last month of Pre-Maintenance? Not necessarily. You might be able, for example, to add a 125 g (4½ oz) serving of brown rice (about

21 grams of Net Carbs and about 108 calories) without experiencing cravings or undue hunger. In that case, you'd likely need to reduce your fat intake slightly. On the other hand, if you have a lower carb tolerance, you'll have to make up that extra calorie demand with a bit more fat, perhaps with half a Hass avocado (less than 2 grams of Net Carbs and 153 calories) or 1 tablespoon almond butter (2.8 grams of Net Carbs and 102 calories). Unless you're eating less than 115–175 g (4–6 oz) of (cooked) protein at each meal, don't increase protein to boost calories. You may have to play a little with this adjustment so as to not overshoot the mark and start gaining weight. Continuing to make entries in your food journal should help you figure out which foods help fill you up without stimulating your appetite unnecessarily.

THE SCOOP ON SUGAR: STARTLING STATS

Toss these statistics from the USDA, Centers for Disease Control, and National Health and Nutrition Examination Survey around the next time someone asks why you've eliminated sugar from your diet.

- Each American consumes an average of 141 g (5 oz) of added sugars a day.
- That adds up to 53 kg (116 lb) of sugar a year. If you're a woman, that might be your goal weight!
- We now consume more than twice as much fructose (fruit sugar), much of it in the form of high-fructose glucose syrup, than we did 30 years ago.
- It's estimated that half of Americans drink one sweetened fizzy drink a day, and 5 per cent have four or more – yes, in one day!
- On average, Americans eat a total of 30 teaspoons a day of added sugar in one form or another.
- The American Heart Association calls for an upper limit of 200 calories a day from added sugars. Which is more astounding, that a major health organisation is this permissive or that most Americans consume far more than this amount?

NO WAY BACK

Here's a question I often hear from Atkins followers: "Now that I've lost weight, why can't I go back to my old way of eating but just be more moderate?" You're welcome to try, but I have to warn you that it's unlikely to work. You've learned that controlling your carb intake makes your body burn primarily fat for energy, which produces that wonderful side effect of moderating your appetite. Return to your old way of eating, and you'll be right back on the blood-sugar roller coaster, experiencing peaks and dips in your energy levels, which leads to overeating. Once more, Lifetime Maintenance is just that – a way of eating that you can sustain and which will maintain your healthy weight. The price you have to pay is small: continue to abstain from added sugar and refined grains, as well as anything that acts as a trigger food. Fortunately, there are so many tasty alternatives that this really isn't difficult, as we'll discuss in the next chapter.

AS TIME GOES BY

Perhaps you're in your forties or older and until recently never had to worry about your weight. Or perhaps you're in your twenties or thirties and assume that now you've slimmed down, you have it made. But things change, and your metabolism may be one of those things. That's why it's a good idea to understand that at some future date you may need to adjust your carb intake up or down in order to continue to maintain your weight. This may result simply from the passage of years, but here are a few other possible reasons to recalibrate:

- You may need to dial your daily Net Carb count down if:
    - An injury sidelines you for a few months.
    - A change in career puts you behind a desk eight hours a day.
    - You're prescribed a drug that slows your metabolism.
    - You enter menopause.

- You may need to dial your daily Net Carb count up if:
    - You take up a vigorous sport such as running or tennis.
    - You move to a fourth-floor flat with no lift.
    - You're chasing after a toddler all day long.

Another very real possibility if you're a young woman is that you'll become pregnant. In this happy event, it's perfectly okay to continue with the Lifetime Maintenance phase of Atkins.

TAKING A BREAK

You may find yourself occasionally in a situation where you need to back off a bit on your low-carb lifestyle for a week or so. Perhaps you're visiting your new in-laws or travelling to another country where you'll be a guest in a private home. In either case, it could be impolite to not eat much of what's put on your plate. Or maybe you're in a new job and have to spend a week in training at the corporate office with all eyes on you. The best way to deal with such a situation is to plan ahead, perhaps by cutting down on your carbs for a week or two before. Also, be sure not to use such a situation as an excuse to pig out on puddings and other problematic foods. Finally, get back in gear immediately upon your return. Here are some more tips:

- At buffets, comply with your Atkins lifestyle, passing up white bread, white rice, gravy made with flour, and other obviously high-carb foods.
- In lieu of juice at breakfast, ask if fruit is available.
- Go easy on alcohol, which can interfere with your food inhibitions.
- Share puddings, have a small bite only, or ask for fruit instead.
- Pack some nuts and/or Atkins bars to keep your appetite under control between meals.
- Don't bore people by talking about how you usually eat.

TROUBLESHOOTING IN PHASE 4

Say you've gained 1.8 kg (4 lb) and want to deal with the situation before it gets any more serious. Simply pare roughly 10 grams of Net Carbs a day from your intake until you return to your goal weight.

Give or take a couple of grams, here are some candidates for subtraction:

- ½ banana
- 150 g (5½ oz) watermelon balls
- ½ large grapefruit
- 2 carrots
- ½ baked potato
- 65 g (2¼ oz) beetroot
- ½ small sweet potato
- 115 g (4 oz) cooked porridge
- 60 g (2¼ oz) brown rice
- 1 slice wholemeal bread
- 35 g (1¼ oz) lentils
- 25 g (1 oz) shelled edamame
- 25 g (1 oz) chickpeas
- 225 g (8 oz) plain yoghurt made with whole milk.

FREQUENTLY ASKED QUESTIONS

We all want to believe that once we've turned over a new leaf, the book stays open to that page. Now that you've reached your goal weight, you surely intend to stay there. But planning to do something and actually doing it aren't always the same. Let's look at some questions that frequently come up at this point in the programme.

Q. What if my carb tolerance never goes above 50 grams of Net Carbs a day?
A. There's tremendous variation in how many carbs individuals can consume and still maintain their weight. Men have more muscle mass and therefore typically a higher metabolism, as do younger people. Hormonal issues also play a role. If you're sedentary, it's worth starting to work out. If you already exercise, increase your level of intensity and/or frequency to see if you can raise your carb tolerance level.

Q. I've been maintaining my weight nicely for several months. Can I occasionally have some of my old faves without upsetting the applecart?
A. Of course you can have a slice of cake at your kid's birthday party, for example, but plan for such occurrences, if possible, by cutting back on carbs for a day or two beforehand. If you find yourself

constantly pushing the limits, however, there's a good risk that your occasional foray into the world of sweetened drinks or eating a bag of crisps on the way home from the supermarket could become a habit. The real risk isn't regaining a bit of weight so much as losing the appetite control that Atkins provides.

Q. I've found that I can eat some sugary foods without gaining weight. Can I keep eating them?
A. Your metabolism may allow you to do so without regaining weight, but as you've read in earlier chapters, added sugar is empty of real nutrients and has been implicated in the rise of obesity and diabetes. Eating such foods also displaces the nutritious vegetables and other wholefoods that are relatively low in carbs. Keep eating these sugary foods and you may find yourself on a slippery slope.

Q. What should I do when I occasionally succumb to temptation and eat an inappropriate food?
A. First of all, don't beat yourself up about it and then use that as an excuse to pig out for the rest of the day. The next day, simply return to following Phase 4 at your appropriate level of carb intake.

Q. On a two-week holiday, I gained back almost 4.5 kg (10 lb) eating all sorts of foods I know I shouldn't have. How do I get back on track ASAP?
A. Being off your own turf and eating out day after day can disrupt your usual routines. The moment you get home, drop down 20 grams of Net Carbs from your usual amount. If a week at this level doesn't do the trick, return to Phase 2 until you achieve your goal weight again.

Q. After six months of maintaining my new weight, I fell off the wagon. How do I repair the damage?
A. Stress at home or work, losing your job, ending a relationship, or countless other changes in your life could push you back into your old habits. First and foremost, don't beat yourself up about it. You know how to lose the weight and how fragile that loss is. Return to Phase 2 until you're in control of your cravings, then gradually move through the phases until you achieve and maintain your goal weight.

CAN YOU REMAIN SLIM FOREVER?

That's a tough question, but one that must be asked. How can you beat the odds I mentioned in the beginning of this chapter? Take this quiz to get a handle on whether you're vulnerable to regaining that excess weight.

1. Have you gained, lost, and regained weight in the past?

   Yes ___ No ___

2. Were you in a hurry to lose weight so you could eat your old favourite foods?

   Yes ___ No ___

3. Do you eat to soothe yourself when you're depressed or under stress?

   Yes ___ No ___

4. Do you still crave sugary or starchy junk foods?

   Yes ___ No ___

5. Do you live with someone who doesn't support your new way of eating?

   Yes ___ No ___

6. Do you enjoy the foods you can eat on Atkins?

   Yes ___ No ___

7. Have you moved through the four phases of Atkins?

   Yes ___ No ___

8. Have you discarded habits, such as eating in front of the telly, that contributed to your weight gain?

   Yes ___ No ___

9. Do you eat regular meals?

   Yes ___ No ___

10. Have you established a physical fitness regime?

    Yes ___ No ___

If you answered yes to several of the first five questions, you could be heading for trouble. Ditto if you responded no to a few of the second five questions. This book has laid out a programme that makes Atkins a sustainable way of eating. If your answers make you concerned that you may be vulnerable to regaining lost weight, review the book to renew your commitment to maintaining the new you.

This test is not meant to discourage you. Rather, I want to encourage you to make Atkins your lifestyle. In the next two chapters, we'll look at how to incorporate Atkins meals into your life whether you're at home or away, as well as explore lots of great new products that make it easier than ever to eliminate empty carbs from your meals.

Now meet Natalie L., who has done just that and gone from wearing a UK size 30 (US size 28) to a UK size 4 (US size 1)! By changing her way of eating, she also was able to dodge her family history of diabetes.

ELEVEN YEARS AND GOING STRONG

VITAL STATS

Daily Net Carb intake:
  60 grams
Age: 37
Height: 168 cm (5 ft 6 in)

Before weight: 172 kg
  (27 st 1 lb)
After weight: 54 kg (8 st 6 lb)
Lost: 118 kg (260 lb)

Like all too many women, Natalie L. had been overweight since she was a teenager and had tried multiple weight-loss programmes without success. And like many other mothers, her pregnancies had aggravated the problem. Being at risk for diabetes didn't help either. But all that was more than a decade ago. Today, the Grayson, Georgia resident is full of health and energy and is less than one-third of her pre-Atkins weight. Natalie fills in the details.

Diabetes runs in my family, and I was diagnosed as pre-diabetic when I was 17. I was told to avoid sugar and other high-carb foods, but I resisted that advice. After all, my favourite foods were ice cream and fried anything. In my family a vegetable was a french fry! Both my parents are overweight and take loads of medications. When we were growing up I was always the funny, chubby one and my sister was the thin, pretty one.

In 2002, when my second son was about 8 months old, I knew I had to make a change. I was desperate to finally find something that worked so that I could feel better and keep up with both my babies. I found an Atkins book in a used-book shop and figured I had nothing to lose but the fat. I felt terrible for the first two weeks. Now I realise I was not getting enough salt. I'd grown up on southern cooking, washing down deep-fried food with Diet Coke! But soon I felt amazing.

My husband had said that we could have another baby if I lost 45 kg (100 lb), which was a big motivator. It took me about nine months to reach that goal, and I got pregnant shortly thereafter. I talked to my doctor about staying on Atkins during the pregnancy and he said that was fine as long as I moved beyond Induction and ate more vegetables. He was much happier with my being 45 kg (100 lb) lighter and doing Atkins than eating double cheeseburgers and french fries, as I had with the last two pregnancies. This time I gained only 3.6 kg (8 lb), and a day after the birth of my third son, I weighed less than I did before I'd become pregnant.

I went back to Induction afterwards to lose the rest of the weight. Its strictness gave me the self-control I needed. I now wear a US size 0 or 1, a major change from my old size 28! Until I lost the weight I'd never realised that I had a small frame. Today my blood sugar and blood pressure are normal, as is my cholesterol. Four years after I'd lost the weight, I was diagnosed with coeliac disease. It was far easier for me than it is for most people to avoid foods with gluten in them because I was already living the Atkins lifestyle.

The control thing was huge for me. Having two babies within 21 months of each other meant that my life was all about everyone else. Atkins lets me take control of my body and my life. When I got married I was only 20. My now ex-husband is a police officer and he used to control what we ate, when we went to the supermarket, and even what I wore. He wasn't happy with the new independent me and didn't like all the attention I was getting. And losing weight made me realise that everything that was wrong with our marriage wasn't my fault. We divorced three years ago and I remarried a year later. My new husband eats the way I do with one exception: no way is he giving up his beer!

We're both very active. He plays tennis and I work out every single day. I joined a 24-hour gym about a month after I started Atkins. I would go after the kids were in bed so that no one would see my fat butt! I started walking on a treadmill and later switched to a better gym, and now I have a gym in the house. I find I do best at about 60 grams of Net Carbs a day. If I go any higher, my skin breaks out and I get headaches. I still have a carb counter on my phone. My weight varies within a 2.2 kg (5-lb) range and I can dial it down if necessary.

Today I'm an estate agent and executive assistant, a job I never could have done when I was obese. It's still hard to see people who can eat everything, but nothing tastes good enough to be worth becoming the "fat girl" again. Now I know that I will live to see my boys grow up.

MAKE IT EASY

When we go on holiday, I take a tape measure to make sure I'm "behaving" in case I can't weigh myself. —NL

PART III

IT'S ALL ABOUT FOOD

CHAPTER 9

IT'S EASY TO EAT AT HOME

Which statement best describes you?

- I love to cook.
- I hate to cook.
- I have no time to cook.
- I cook occasionally.
- I do my real cooking on the weekends.

Or are you a combination of several of the above, depending on your mood, day, workload, and other commitments? If you're like me, you may enjoy cooking when entertaining friends and family but not the pressure to cook every night. Or perhaps you're worried that making food suitable for Atkins is more complicated than "regular" cooking. (If someone else does most of the cooking in your family, share this chapter with him or her.)

Regardless of your attitude towards cooking, I can assure you that it's perfectly possible to get tasty, low-carb meals suitable for the whole family on the table with a minimum of time and fuss. Whether you're looking for quick and easy recipes, no-cook meals, make-in-advance meals, cook-while-you're-away meals, or cook-once-and-eat-twice meals, you'll find multiple solutions to the eternal problem of what to have for dinner tonight. Similar options apply to breakfast and lunch. Recipes begin on page 211 and are coded to indicate whether they contain a minimal number of ingredients, have a prep time of 20 minutes or less, are make-in-advance meals, or can be made in a slow cooker.

MEALS FOR THE WHOLE FAMILY

Let's dispel one myth. There's no need to cook two separate meals, one for you and another for the rest of the family. Likewise, if you live alone, you can serve visitors the same foods you're eating without occasioning any strange looks. That's because Atkins-style cooking isn't that different from "regular" cooking. The key difference is the avoidance of certain ingredients, such as sugar, refined grains, and vegetable oil, and of breading and deep-frying food.

Basically, you simply subtract (or substitute) one or more items from the menu that the rest of the family will be eating. Here are some examples of how to feed the family while complying with your own needs with a minimum of extra work. And when a family meal is really high in carbs, Atkins products, including the low-carb pasta, can be a lifesaver.

THEM	YOU
Scrambled eggs and bacon with toast	Scrambled eggs and bacon with sliced tomatoes
Hot dogs on rolls, baked beans, cucumber sticks	Hot dogs, sauerkraut, cucumber sticks
Roast chicken, steamed spinach, baked sweet potatoes	Roast chicken, steamed spinach, celery sticks with blue cheese dressing
Cereal with blueberries and milk	An Atkins Advantage bar and blueberries*
Beef burger on a bun; side salad, steamed green beans, chips	Beef burger; side salad, steamed green beans

*In Phase 2.

ALL IN THE FAMILY

Dinner is the most likely time that the family eats together. Your decision to go on Atkins may throw a curveball into family dynamics at first, until it becomes clear that Atkins is simply a healthy way to eat. Some advice:

- *If you're the primary cook:* Assure your partner that his or her meal preferences will be honoured. For example, if pasta or another starchy dish is a must in your partner's book, you might make grilled salmon, a salad, and pasta for dinner and simply pass on the pasta. And really, how much trouble is it to boil the water for pasta, pop some potatoes in the oven, or steam rice in a microwave packet? If it preserves domestic harmony as you lose weight, why not?

- *If your mate is the chef:* Explain that there's not going to be any extra work. Any meal is fine as long as there is a protein source such as chicken or burgers without a starchy sauce, plus a vegetable and/or salad. If macaroni cheese or another high-carb meal is on the menu, simply swap vegetables in a starchy sauce for a salad.

FAMILY POLITICS

Changing the way you eat can make your nearest and dearest uncomfortable. A conversation with your partner and/or kids can usually eliminate any concerns. And then there's the matter of your extended family. Let's take these one by one.

- *Significant others.* If you're lucky, your partner understands your reasons for deciding to lose weight and respects your choice of Atkins. She or he may even be joining you on the programme. On the other hand, your partner might feel threatened by your decision, particularly if she or he is also overweight. Or your partner may simply not understand how cutting carbs and eating healthy fats can result in dramatic weight loss. If so, suggest reading Chapter 1 of this book. Make sure not to disparage his or her weight or knowledge of nutrition. Also make it clear that you're not asking permission to do Atkins. Simply explain that you believe this is right for you and you'd appreciate understanding.

- *Kids.* If parents are relaxed and comfortable with the offerings at mealtime, the fact that you're doing Atkins should be a non-issue. Obviously younger kids may react, if at all, differently than teens. Assure kids that family meals won't change; you just might not eat everything they eat. As long as the way you eat doesn't threaten them, kids should be fine. They might even follow your lead as they see you snacking on nuts and eating lots of vegetables and simply prepared protein dishes. Never nag your children about eating too much of something or not enough of another food, and never bring up their weight in the context of a meal.

- *Extended family.* Eating habits can carry a lot of emotional freight in some families. Your sister, mother, mother-in-law, or grandmother could feel threatened by your decision to start on Atkins, especially if she is also overweight. In cultures with strong culinary traditions, your new way of eating, sans pasta or potatoes, for example, could make your relatives feel you're rejecting family traditions. Reassure them that you're not impugning their apple pie, calzones, beef burritos, or Yorkshire pudding. Rather, losing weight is something you need to do to feel good about yourself. Explain that that's why you won't be eating a particular food (even just a taste) at the next family dinner. Make it clear that you respect their choices and trust that they will respect yours. By all means, don't act superior (a risk for new converts of any sort) or challenge their culinary approach.

Now let's get down to how to make it easier to get food on the table. We'll cover the gamut from meals you can toss together from store-cupboard staples and leftovers to main-dish salads, quick stir-fries and slow-cooker dishes, and more. Among these choices, you're sure to find some that suit your culinary preferences and cooking style.

NO-TIME-TO-SHOP MEALS

Your first objective is to always have Atkins-appropriate food available. You can find all the basics you'll need in a supermarket. If you cook regularly, you probably already have a number of those basics on hand. You don't necessarily have to have everything in the kitchen at all times. For example, if you shop weekly, you may not need more than one or two protein sources in the freezer. But once you fill your fridge, freezer, and store cupboards (and restock regularly) with acceptable foods, you'll never find yourself with "nothing to eat".

NO-COOK MEALS

Sometimes I'm just too whacked to make dinner after work, but the last thing I want to do is eat out. I'd much rather chill out at home in my track suit and slippers. I'm sure you often feel the same way. Of course, takeaway is an option, but it's almost as pricey as eating at a restaurant. What to do?

Fortunately, with salad bars, delis, and a whole array of ready-to-serve products at the supermarket, you have another set of options. The granddaddy of such offerings is the rotisserie-roasted chicken. After a short stop, you'll be able to assemble a no-cook meal in minutes. A word of caution: many foods in delis and salad bars are full of high-carb ingredients, so ask questions, read labels, and avoid meats cured with nitrates or made with bread crumbs and other fillers, starchy sauces, and salads with added sugar.

From the Deli

- Rotisserie-roasted chicken; chicken, tuna, egg, whitefish, or prawn salad; smoked salmon; grilled, roasted, or poached chicken
- Ham, pastrami, salt beef, salami,* roast or smoked turkey, grilled chicken breast
- Sauerkraut, gherkins, pickled green beans, pickled mushrooms, cucumber salad, coleslaw, olives

Avoid products with nitrates.

From the Salad Bar

- Grilled, roasted, or baked turkey, salmon, tuna, and chicken; grilled or steamed prawns; tofu; hard-boiled eggs
- Grilled, roasted, or steamed broccoli, asparagus, cauliflower, green beans, and other foundation vegetables (without problematic sauces)
- Salad leaves, tomatoes, avocado, and other salad vegetables
- Olives, hummus (in Phase 2), baba ganoush (aubergine dip)
- Berries and melon chunks (in Phase 2); additional fruit (in Phase 3 or 4)
- Nuts, seeds, crumbled bacon, grated cheese
- Feta cheese, Cheddar cheese, etc.
- Vinaigrette, blue cheese, or ranch dressing
- What to avoid: meats and fish with starchy sauces, croutons, crunchy noodles, bean salads (unless you're in Phase 2), pasta salads, and other composed salads with off-limits ingredients; imitation crab (surimi); sushi; stuffed vine leaves; crackers.

From the Supermarket

In addition to the ingredients listed above, check out:

- Tinned salmon or tuna
- Bagged coleslaw and washed and bagged salad mixes
- Trimmed and cut-up vegetables and fruits.

Put it All Together

Here are a few no-cook combos for busy nights:

- Grilled chicken with green beans and salad from the salad bar
- A bagged salad topped with a tuna steak and asparagus
- Salt beef with sauerkraut and cucumber salad
- Smoked turkey over coleslaw with ranch dressing
- Sliced ham and antipasto items such as marinated artichoke hearts, roasted sweet peppers, mushrooms, olives, and feta cheese
- Grated courgettes topped with a salmon steak and pesto.

WHEN A SALAD IS PLENTY

A robust salad can be the main attraction rather than just an accompaniment to a meal. Plus, most salads can also be prepared in minutes. Our recipe developer has come up with six winners, starting on page 236, all of which are suitable for all phases of Atkins:

- Chipotle Prawn Salad
- Grilled Chicken and Marinated Kale Salad
- Buffalo Chicken Salad
- Turkey Enchilada Salad
- Crisp Lettuce Wedge with Sliced Flank Steak
- All-season Caprese Salad with Prosciutto

You can also check atkins.com for more main dish salad recipes.

MEALS ON THE DOUBLE

Next up are meals you can prepare with minimal fuss thanks to a host of products ready to heat up in the microwave or on the hob. You'll find such time-savers as you prowl the supermarket. Unfortunately, some prepared foods often involve a trade-off between certain ingredients and convenience, so read food labels carefully.

- Skip the sea of fish fingers, fish cakes, and other battered or breaded prepared fish dishes and seek out the few acceptable alternatives, including grilled tilapia, salmon, and pollock.
- You can also find several kinds of frozen fish fillets in individual-portion vacuum-sealed bags. Remove from the freezer in the morning to defrost in the fridge. Unbreaded frozen prawns, scallops, and calamari also come in handy for quick stir-fries.
- Look for frozen tilapia, prawns, and other fish dishes that cook in a marinade of lemon juice and other seasonings inside parchment parcels (you can make these from baking parchment).
- Chicken breasts, individually packaged burgers, lamb or pork chops, and sausages are other good quick-cooking protein options. As with fish, pair with a cooked vegetable and a salad.
- Top grilled pork chops or meatballs with a bottled tomato sauce. Or serve chicken, turkey breast, or veal with a bottled carbonara sauce. Look for products without added sugar such as Bella Vita low

carb sauces, Jok n Al sauces and Walden Farms sauces (available at www.avidlite.com or www.lowcarbmegastore.com.) (Not all products from these brands have no added sugar; read labels carefully.)

- Simmer sauces let you put together a curry in minutes. Simply heat leftover chicken or another meat, prawns, or packaged chunks of grilled or roasted chicken or turkey in the sauce. Add some frozen vegetables and serve over brown rice (or spaghetti squash, bean sprouts, or grated courgettes if you're not eating wholegrains).

- Frozen vegetables in microwave steamer bags are a speedy option and eliminate having to wash another pan. Just be sure to purchase those without sauces made with starches and/or added sugar.

MAKE IT EASY

To save on washing up, bake individual fish fillets or chicken breasts in a tightly sealed foil packet placed on a baking tray. Before sealing the packet, add a pat of butter, some thinly sliced vegetables, and seasonings. Bake in the oven at 200°C (400°F) for 20–25 minutes.

SAVE AS YOU SLIM DOWN

There are countless inexpensive low-carb options, and the first step to keeping a lid on costs is to plan your meals and recipes for the week. Having meal ingredients to hand prevents you from having to make last-minute trips to the supermarket, hitting a fast-food place, or ordering a takeaway for dinner. Here are more ways to start saving:

- *Choose cheaper cuts of meat.* There's no need to eat pricey beef fillet. Flank and rump contain more fat, making them flavourful, juicy, and well suited to slow-cooked dishes such as stews, soups, and roasts. Lamb shanks, ham steaks, rib and shoulder pork chops, and pork, chicken, or turkey sausages are other budget-friendly choices. Buy meat in bulk when certain cuts are on sale and freeze in single or family-size portions.

- *Pass on chicken pieces.* Whole chickens are almost always less expensive per kilo than packaged pieces. Joint a whole chicken or roast a whole bird for several meals over the course of a week.
- *Go fish.* Don't assume that salmon, cod, prawns and scallops are the only way to go. Tilapia, sea bass, sardines, mackerel, and mussels are less pricey options.
- *Think beyond fish, poultry, and meat.* Eggs, legumes (pulses), and tofu and other soy-based foods can stand in for the usual protein sources. Turkey mince is another economical choice. Vegetarian protein crumbles or sausage can substitute for beef mince in chilli and other recipes.
- *Bag the bag.* Washed, chopped, and bagged salad leaves are a time saver but are always more expensive than a head of lettuce or other greens.
- Shop in bulk. Some supermarkets now have bulk food sections where you can save on nuts, seeds, pulses, and wholegrains.
- *Cheaper by the litre.* Instead of purchasing expensive bottled or canned soft drinks, make big batches of low-carb lemonade, iced tea, and coffee drinks using an acceptable sweetener. Or flavour water with a squeeze of lemon or lime or a few sprigs of mint. You'll be helping the planet while pinching pennies.

COOK ONCE, EAT TWICE

One way to save both time and money is to double or even triple recipes and freeze some, perhaps in individual portions for future meals. Or let a dish such as our Deep-Dish Sausage and Cauliflower Pizza (page 224) or Cheesy Chicken and Green Bean Sauté (page 225) do double duty as lunch the following day. Stews and slow-cooker dishes such as Slow Cooker Pork and Salsa Verde Parcels (page 228) are great candidates for doubling the recipe, as are soups such as Salmon Mushroom Chowder (page 249) and No-Bean Chicken Chilli (page 245). You can also "remodel" leftover vegetables, for example, by adding stock and some leftover chicken or meat to make a hearty soup suitable for lunch on its own.

Experienced cooks know that for all its impressive presentation, making a roast beef, pork loin, chicken, or leg of lamb is easy to do – set the timer and forget about it. That weekend dish then pays dividends for the rest of the week. It's a time-honoured way to get several meals out of one purchase and make the most of leftovers. A large roast chicken, for instance, could provide chicken salad for lunch the next day, chicken curry the following evening, and stir-fry with Asian vegetables later in the week. If you're feeling industrious, you can even use the carcass to make chicken stock. The leftovers from beef, pork, and lamb roasts provide just as many opportunities for creativity. Once you open your mind to the possibilities, you'll learn to love your leftovers.

SPEEDY STIR-FRIES

You don't need a wok to put together a tasty one-dish meal – a deep-sided frying pan will do the job. Technically, stir-frying takes place at a higher temperature than sautéing, but both techniques require cutting food up into small pieces and frequent turning and stirring to hasten the cooking process. Cutting up ingredients requires the most time, but you can take a shortcut by purchasing fresh vegetables already cut up. Most supermarkets offer them, or pick them up at a salad bar. Or use frozen vegetables. Nor are Asian seasonings a must; try stir-fries that draw from other cuisines as well. A few possibilities:

- Asian Beef Stir-Fry (page 226)
- Cheesy Chicken and Green Bean Sauté (page 225)

From atkins.com:

- Creamy Beef and Mixed Mushroom Stir-fry
- Prawn and Bok Choy Stir-Fry
- Beef and Broccoli Stir-Fry
- Stir-Fried Scallops with Asparagus

You'll find that it's easy to modify the recipes in this book by swapping one ingredient for another. So if a recipe calls for pork tenderloin, the same amount of chicken breast or beef sirloin can usually make a fine substitute. Likewise, if a recipe calls for asparagus and it's not in season or too expensive, green beans or broccoli can stand in.

A SLOW BUT STEADY SILENT HELPER

It may seem counterintuitive, but a slow cooker may be just what you need to get meals on the table fast. If you work outside the home or are ferrying your kids here, there, and everywhere, it almost allows you to be in two places at once. Slow cooking intensifies flavours and tenderises meats, making it ideal for cheaper cuts. In addition to delicious soups and stews, recipes for casseroles, curries, and roasts are easily adapted to the slow cooker. Here's a week's worth of easy recipes that lend themselves to this way of cooking.

- Slow Cooker Pork and Salsa Verde (page 228)
- No-Bean Chicken Chilli (page 245)
- Salmon Mushroom Chowder (page 249)
- Taco Soup (page 246)

At atkins.com:

- Hearty Beef Stew
- Lamb Stew
- Lemon Thyme Tenderloin with Roasted Vegetables

A SMARTPHONE IN THE KITCHEN

Once upon a time if you had a great meal at a restaurant you might rave about it on the phone to a friend the next day. Or if you turned out a particularly yummy dish, you could share your excitement by scanning and sharing the recipe. But today you can snap a picture with your smartphone, boast about your success on countless websites, or simply text your mum or another good cook for advice on a recipe or an ingredient. Many mobile apps, including the app you can download at atkins.com, also make it easier to prepare meals by helping you make up a shopping list, "clip" coupons, compare prices, and plan meals — all in one place.

THE SCOOP ON SUGAR: SWEET AND SAVOURY SUBSTITUTES

You expect to find added sugar in sweets, but it all too often turns up in savoury sauces and other products where you would least expect it. Fortunately, many large food companies now manufacture sugar-free or no-sugar-added versions of their brands, including those listed below. Speciality companies have also stepped up to the plate with sugar-free versions of favourite foods. All of the following replacements are acceptable in Phase 1. Some, such as Heinz products, can be found in the supermarket. Others may need to be ordered online (see "Low-Carb Resources", on page 184, for URLs). *Heinz do offer reduced sugar but not sugar free.*

INSTEAD OF:	TRY THIS:
Starbucks Flavoured Coffee Drinks	Coffee plus Da Vinci Sugar-free Syrup
Marshmallows	La Nouba Sugar-Free Marshmallows
Hard Sweets	AJ's Sugar-free Sweets
Wine Gums	De Bron Wine Gums
Barbecue Sauce	Walden Farms Barbecue Sauce
Heinz Ketchup	Heinz Reduced Sugar Ketchup
	Walden Farms Ketchup
Chilli Pepper Sauce	Jok n Al Chilli Pepper Sauce
Chocolate Syrup	Da Vinci Sugar-free Chocolate Syrup
Del Monte Cocktail/Seafood Sauce	Jok n Al Sugar-free Cocktail Sauce

SWAP THE SAUCE

Are you in a rut serving the same five or six dishes week after week: "If it's Wednesday, it must be pork chops?" It's understandable that saving time is high on your list of priorities, but that needn't mean mealtime mono-tony. Easy-to-make sauces, marinades, and dressings can spice up plain fish, chicken, or meat dishes. Find several sauces you like and use them on a variety of protein choices. Add a vegetable and perhaps a side salad, and dinner can be on the table in minutes. Use the five sauces in the recipe section on a variety of protein sources and add a phase-appropriate vegetable or salad to each combo, and you won't have to repeat yourself for months. Plus you'll find many more sauce-and-main meal combinations in the Atkins recipe database.

SAUCE	PROTEIN SOURCE	SUITABLE SAUCES
1. Lemon Tartare	Chicken breast	1, 2, 3, 4, 5
2. Chipotle BBQ Sauce	Pork chops	2, 3, 4, 5
3. Creamy Sweet Soya	Turkey sausages	2, 3, 4, 5
4. Parmesan-Garlic White Sauce	Flank steak	2, 3, 4, 5
5. Spicy, Chunky Tomato	Beef burgers	1, 2, 4, 5
	Salmon	1, 2, 3, 4
	Prawns	1, 2, 3, 4, 5
	Tilapia	1, 2, 3, 4, 5
	Ham steak	2, 3, 4
	Tofu cubes	2, 3, 4

CLASSICS, ATKINS-STYLE

Foods such as mashed potatoes, fajitas, beef stroganoff, and chips seem to be an integral part of our DNA! These classics are sky high in carbs and we know we shouldn't eat them – or at least only on special occasions – but they're darn near irresistible. Fortunately, there are ways to fool your taste buds with persuasive substitutes. Look at the comparable servings of a low-carb alternative to the classic dish to make your decision easy:

CLASSIC	ATKINS ALTERNATIVE	REDUCTION IN NET CARBS
Mashed potato	Mashed cauliflower	78%
Chips	Baked sweet potato "fries"	66%
Chips	Turnip fries	87%
Chilli con carne	No-Bean Chicken Chilli*	55%
Beef stroganoff on egg noodles	Beef stroganoff on shredded courgettes	90%
Beef stroganoff on egg noodles	Beef stroganoff on Atkins low carb penee or fusilli	53%
Spaghetti and meatballs	Spaghetti squash and meatballs	90%

*Recipe included in this book.

LOW-CARB RESOURCES

You can, of course, order Atkins Advantage bars and shakes, Day Break bars, Endulge bars and Atkins penne or fusilli pasta at buyatkins.co.uk, as well as find them in retail outlets. The following companies manufacture or sell other Atkins-friendly foods you may want to explore. Some are available at supermarkets and discount clubs; others may need to be ordered online. Many sites have a store locator feature. This is hardly a complete list, but it should give you an idea of the range of low-carb products available.

- AJ's low-carb sweets, including Cola Fizz, Bakewell Tart and Mint Humbugs *
- Dietimeal sugar-free shakes and puddings*
- Ciao Carb biscuits*
- Linwoods Organic Flaxseed and Tiana Coconut Flour (hollandandbarrett.com)
- Dixie Diner pizza mix and Carbophobia Bread mix*
- Miss Meringue sugar-free flavoured meringues (missmeringue.com)
- DaVinci Gourmet sugar-free syrups and sauces*
- Sweetbird sugar-free coffee flavourings (nextdaycoffee.co.uk)

- Butcher's pork scratchings, Kallo mini rice cakes (Carbgenie.com)
- Walden Farm's sugar-free sauces (amazon.co.uk)
- Fresh baked low-carb bread & rolls*
- Cavalier Cinnamon Crisps*
- La Nouba sugar-free preserves, marshmallows, and a chocolate hazelnut spread that tastes like Nutella, all made in Belgium (lanouba.be)
- Stute sugar-free jam (amazon.co.uk)
- Joseph's low-carb bread and tortilla wraps*
- Aunt Bessie no added sugar custard (avidlite.co.uk)
- Alpro unsweetened soya milk (alpro.com)
- Balance no added sugar chocolate spread*
- Carbthin zero carb baking mix*

* All available on lowcarbmegastore.com

THE SCOOP ON SUGAR: NATURAL, BUT STILL SUGAR

Mother Nature produces honey, maple syrup, molasses, and agave syrup, which all boast traces of antioxidants, but all of these still deliver a dense dose of carbs, as you can see below.

PRODUCT	AMOUNT	NET CARBS
Table sugar	1 tablespoon	12.6 g
Agave nectar	25 g (1 oz)	20 g
Honey	1 tablespoon	17 g
Molasses	1 tablespoon	15 g
Maple syrup	1 tablespoon	15 g

BETTER CHOCOLATE CHOICES

Everyone loves chocolate, but most chocolate treats are sugar bombs. Instead, opt for substitutes over old favourites and you'll slash your sugar and carb intake. Put some of these products to the taste test.

HAVE THIS	INSTEAD OF THAT	QUANTITY	DIFFERENCE IN NET CARBS
Atkins Advantage Milk Chocolate Ready to Drink	Chocolate Ice Cream Shake	330 ml	75 g
Atkins Endulge Peanut Caramel bar	Snickers	1 bar	30 g
Atkins Advantage Chocolate Brownie bar	Milky Way	1 bar	34 g
AvidHiPro Chocolate Ice Cream	Chocolate Ice Cream	40 g	21 g
Balance No Added Sugar Chocolate Spread	Nutella	1 tablespoon	9 g

FREQUENTLY ASKED QUESTIONS

Q. Do I have to rewash pre-washed salad leaves?
A. These leaves are a great convenience, but it's still a good idea to rinse and give them a whirl in a salad spinner. Salad leaves usually stay crisp for up to five days when placed in a resealable plastic bag with a damp paper towel.

Q. I know I shouldn't eat them, but I still crave the crunch and saltiness of pretzels and crisps. What do you recommend instead?
A. Actually, there are several alternatives. Rather than buying salted nuts or seeds, you could lightly sprinkle them with salt to moderate the inclination to keep eating them. Air-popped popcorn sprinkled with Parmesan cheese or a bit of seasoned salt is fine in moderation in later phases of Atkins. Low-carb soy and vegetable crisps may also satisfy you.

Q. Now that I'm maintaining my weight, can I have ice cream?
A. An occasional 115 g (4 oz) of ice cream is not going to make you balloon up, but it may be hard to have just a small serving. A better approach is to explore ice creams made without added sugar, including some by Avidlite and Everest Ice. Other frozen low-carb treats include fudge pops, fruit bars, sorbet, and coconut-milk or tofu-based frozen treats, also minus added sugar.

Now that you know how easy it is to put a low-carb meal on the table, it's time to learn how to make dining out just as simple and pleasurable.

As you'll see in the next chapter, as long as you're prepared and know which questions to ask, you should be able to pick and choose from just about any menu, whether it's a Greek diner, fast-food chain, family dining spot, or fine restaurant. But first I want to introduce you to Joe Z., a tae kwon do champion and trainer who had, nonetheless, let himself become obese. More than 91 kg (200 lb) lighter after adopting the Atkins Diet, Joe has rediscovered his self-esteem and found his mission in life: to inspire others to adopt a healthy lifestyle.

FROM DENIAL TO ACCOUNTABILITY

VITAL STATS

Daily Net Carb intake:
   60 grams
Age: 52
Height: 188 cm (6 ft 2 in)

Before weight: 199 kg
   (31 st 4 lb)
After weight: 104 kg
   (16 st 5 lb)
Weight lost: 95 kg (208 lb)

Imagine tipping the scale at 200 kg (440 lb) while teaching tae kwon do in your own school! Six years ago Sacramento, California resident Joe Z. was living a life full of such contradictions. He was also suffering constant back and knee pain and taking Ibuprofen and other painkillers, along with cortisone injections, to try to alleviate it. And by the way, that weight is an estimate, since Joe couldn't find a set of scales that went that high! What is a fact is that he's now almost half the size he was. Let's hear it from Joe.

I was in complete denial. I grew up in a Latino family eating lots of beans, rice, and tortillas. I had been a jock in high school, playing on the football, tennis, and wrestling teams. I was always a big guy, and somehow I convinced myself that my 142-cm (56-inch) waist wasn't that different from its former 91 cm (36 inches). When I was teaching a class, I'd look in the mirror and see a thin person. Then in 2007 I was watching a video of the tae kwon do world championship and I saw someone familiar on an escalator in front of one of my students. I suddenly realised that huge old guy was me!

I had been so unhappy and depressed that all I wanted to do was hide and eat. When I wasn't working, I'd barricade myself in the bedroom with snack food and watch television, which certainly didn't help my marriage. I often asked myself, "How could I have gotten so out of shape?" Of course, my eating habits were terrible. I'd either skip breakfast or hit a drive-in for fast food. Lunch was two main meals and two sets of sides, followed by an afternoon snack and an energy drink. I'd drink sugary, fizzy drinks all day and then go by a fast-food place on the way home for dinner.

I could no longer do the simple kicks to demonstrate techniques to my students. At night, I snored like a freight train.

After glimpsing myself on that video, I finally decided to take control of my life. Previously, I'd tried fen-phen, Weight Watchers, Medifast, and Nutrisystem, among others. I'd lose 22.5 kg (50 lb), feel good, and then gain back 32 kg (70 lb). I started my weight-loss journey on 1 January 2008, as part of a New Year's resolution after reading the Atkins books.

I stayed in Induction for about six months, during which time my youngest daughter, who was then a senior in high school, was my Atkins buddy. During this time, my marriage fell apart, but I stayed with Atkins for two and a half years, ultimately losing 100 kg (220 lb).

Six years later I continue to avoid sugar, pasta, grains, white potatoes, and fizzy drinks. I drink tea without sweetener. If I eat fast food, it's a burger without a bun. When I go to a restaurant I have a salad with chicken or meat and bring my own dressing. I love to cook, and everything I make is low in carbs. My portions are about the size of my fist. Speaking of fists, when I look at my hands today, I don't recognise them. Even my formerly wide feet are now thin. I had no idea how good it could feel to be pain-free and fit into clothes I thought I could never wear. And with my blood pressure at 110/68, my doctor says I'm a new man.

But those aren't even the biggest changes. As the weight came off, my self-esteem improved. My goal has changed from losing weight to becoming as healthy as possible. I've run my first 5-km race and I'm in a weight-training programme. Ironically, now that I'm trying to build muscle I welcome the 5.5 kg (12 lb) I've added! I only wish I'd started weight training earlier to improve muscle tone and help firm up my excess flesh. There are two other huge changes in my life. My second wife, who is a triathlete, was one of my former students. We met when I was plenty big, and when I got down to about 122 kg (270 lb), she asked me out! I've also embarked on a new career as a massage therapist.

In addition to my daughter, my success influenced my boss's mother to go on the Atkins programme. My hope is to inspire other obese people to reach their weight-loss goals. I'm very active on Facebook. Parents of students and former students often ask for advice on how to eat and cook. I meet regularly with a group of over-weight people to talk and work out together. One of the things I tell them is that at some point you have to look in the mirror and say, "I'm the one doing this to myself."

MAKE IT EASY

Don't get obsessed with a certain number. And don't panic when you hit a plateau. I sometimes lost no weight for three weeks at a time. *—JZ*

CHAPTER 10

DINE OUT WITH EASE

Now that you know that Atkins-style eating is no more complicated or time-consuming than putting together other meals, you'll be happy to hear that eating out is just as easy. Much of the advice on how to stay on Atkins on your own turf also applies to dining out. Ditto for meals eaten in the workplace, whether at a company event, in the company canteen, or at your desk. Even when you're on a plane or in a hotel, it's perfectly possible to enjoy an Atkins-friendly meal. To stay in control of just about any food-related situation, it's just a matter of mental preparation and mastering a few techniques.

THE IMPORTANCE OF PLANNING AHEAD

Just as it's essential to have the right foods in your kitchen so you aren't blindsided when mealtime rolls around, planning ahead can be your salvation when it comes to meals in the outside world. Let's look at how that applies to eating in a restaurant, whether it's a white-tablecloth place or a coffee bar.

- *Vet the eatery.* Before you firm up plans or make a reservation, check out the menu online if you can. If the low-carb choices are limited, you may prefer not to put yourself in that situation. No menu online? Check the Yellow Pages under "Restaurants", where menus often appear. Or do a stroll-by and scope out the menu posted in the window. If it's a takeaway place, ask for a copy of the menu for future orders.

- *Know before you go.* Once you decide on a restaurant (or have been invited by someone else), review the menu online. Then and there, decide what to order. When you place your order, don't be swayed by what others are ordering or the specials that the waiter describes in irresistible terms.

- *Eat before you leave home.* This may sound like cleaning the house before the cleaning service arrives, but taking the edge off your hunger puts you and not your low blood sugar in the driver's seat when you sit down to eat. Half an Atkins bar, a chunk of cheese, a few slices of turkey breast, or another snack with protein and healthy fats is usually enough. However, if you're attending a dinner party where the meal may not be served until well after you usually eat, you might be wise to have a light meal, perhaps a salad topped with a protein source.

Your objective, of course, is to stay in control of the situation and not let such occasions become an excuse for falling off the Atkins wagon.

EAT OUT WITHOUT BLOWING IT

Around 7.7 billion informal meals are eaten out in the UK every year. That's 128 meals for every person in the UK. Fortunately, you can eat out almost anywhere, as long as you pick and choose carefully. Regardless of cuisine or price point, all restaurants are in the service business, and making you happy increases the likelihood that you'll return. To become an informed diner:

- *Make your wishes clear.* Be sure the waiting staff understands any modifications you want.
- *Take menu health claims with a large pinch of salt.* There are no standards for the terms "low carb" or "healthy". Plus the latter usually refers to low fat, regardless of how much sugar is in a dish.
- *No sauce, please.* Order a dish prepared without sugar or starches. And steer clear of gravy, which is almost always thickened with flour or cornflour.

- *No breading or batter either.* Inquire about ingredients and cooking techniques. Make sure the main course is roasted, grilled, pan-fried, or poached. Breaded or battered deep-fried dishes may contain harmful trans fats as well as carbs.
- *Downsize supersized portions.* Share a dish or take half home in a doggy bag.
- *Pass on stews.* They're often full of potatoes or other starchy vegetables.
- *Avoid temptation.* Ask for olives or cut-up vegetables in lieu of bread.
- *Double up.* Request a side salad or an additional serving of vegetables instead of the usual rice or potato served with the main course. If your carb tolerance allows, ask for brown rice or another wholegrain.
- *Dress down.* Avoid packaged salad dressings, which are usually full of sugar or corn syrup, and most house dressings. Instead, ask for oil and vinegar (or lemon juice).
- *Have a fallback.* If nothing on the menu seems "safe", ask for a large salad topped with salmon, chicken, or another protein source.
- *End on a low (carb) note.* A bowl of berries with whipping cream or a cheese plate makes a great substitute for a high-carb pudding once you're out of Induction.

RESTAURANT ETIQUETTE

Eating out is about socialising as well as sustenance. Your pals are there to see you, not to get a lecture on how to eat or be made to feel guilty because they're digging into a huge plate of pasta. Likewise, you can get information about ingredients and such from waiting staff without needing to expound on your eating habits. Follow these pointers:

- *Be friendly but firm.* There's no need to tell your companions why you are ordering a Greek salad instead of macaroni cheese, but neither must you help them consume a loaf of Italian bread to be companionable. If asked, simply respond that you had a huge lunch, are cutting down on wheat, or are saving room for your main course. If a friend who knows you're doing Atkins pressures you to share a decadent pudding, remind him or her that you're watching your weight.

- *Treat the waiting staff with patience.* Depending on the type of restaurant and the management style, the staff may or may not be well informed about the ingredients in a dish. If you don't get a satisfactory answer, inquire pleasantly if you can talk to the manager or chef. With so many people suffering from food allergies, many restaurants will modify a dish or eliminate an ingredient on request.

Your objective is always to make the best choices and know what you're eating, not to be cowed into eating something you're not comfortable with. At the same time, the last thing you want to do is make the occasion all about you and your eating habits.

TAKE CONTROL OF THE CONVERSATION

If your low-carb approach to eating provokes your fellow diners, try these gambits. Just be polite and smile nicely as you respond.

He or she says, "Relax, we're out on the town. One little bit of bread" – or pasta, or alcohol, or dessert – "isn't going to kill you."

- Don't respond, "Don't you realise this is a one-way ticket to the blood-sugar roller coaster?"
- Instead say, "Thanks, but I'm watching my carbs right now."

He or she says, "Let's share that chocolate lava cake."

- Don't respond, "It's full of sugar, and sugar might as well be poison."
- Instead say, "I wish I could, but I fear that if I start eating it, I won't be able to stop and there'll be none for you!"

He or she says, "Let's order a couple of pizzas for everyone."

- Don't respond, "Don't you know they're made with white flour, which contains about as many nutrients as the pizza box?"
- Instead say, "You know I love pizza and I love eating with you guys, so go ahead, but I'll order a big salad."

FAST FOOD, YOUR WAY

It can be hard to avoid the major chains when you're on the road, grabbing lunch between appointments, or taking the family out without breaking the bank. Yes, fast food is convenient and inexpensive, but most offerings are full of empty carbs: in the bun, crust, breading, and condiments, and of course in the fries. Plus the beverages and condiments are full of sugar and the portions of everything are enormous. That said, take the trouble to find the options that are more acceptable than others. Some chains boast bunless burgers and other offerings. Almost every major chain, and even some of the regional ones, provide extensive nutritional information on their websites so you know how many carbs are in most offerings. Some even allow you to add or subtract the bun or/and condiments and immediately see the nutritional impact. For example, remove the bun and a Whopper goes from 51 to 3 grams of Net Carbs. In some cases you'll have to calculate Net Carbs by subtracting fibre content. Unfortunately, it's often difficult to tell whether sugar is integral or added, or whether there's sugar in one salad dressing but not another. A few general tips:

- As usual, avoid anything battered, breaded, or deep-fried. Most chicken chains now offer a grilled, or roasted alternative. Pass on fries, baked beans and corn on the cob as well.
- Watch out for sauces and salad dressings that contain added sugar or corn syrup. Your best bets are usually vinaigrette, ranch, and blue cheese dressings.
- Some chains let you order a burger wrapped in lettuce leaves. If not, simply remove the bun and ask for a fork.
- Most chains now offer main-dish salads with ham or chicken.
- However, not every salad is necessarily low in carbs. Check the nutritional profile to be sure.
- Select beverages made with non-caloric sweeteners.

Our suggestions on what to order and what to avoid at five national chains follow. Again, the best approach is to check the menu online, make up your mind before you go, and stick to your guns.

Burger King Again, lose the bun, and most burgers, Whoppers, and the Chicken Royale pass muster. Salads are usually full of high-carb additions, but two exceptions are the Grilled Chicken

Salad and Garden Salad. Be sure to order either with the grilled (not fried) chicken, remove the croutons, and top with low carb dressing. Website: burgerking.co.uk.

KFC offers at least one acceptable dish, the Kentucky Grilled Chicken. Pass on the mashed potatoes, mac n cheese and wedges; instead, have a side of green beans. Website: kfc.com.

McDonald's burgers and cheeseburgers are fine "naked", as is the grilled chicken, the Grilled Chicken and Bacon Salad or Garden Salad with or without grilled chicken, and scrambled eggs and sausage patties. Website: mcdonalds.co.uk.

Pizza Hut Most foods would be unacceptable here except for the large selection of salad vegetables, including lettuce, tomatoes, cucumber, grapes, peppers, jalapeños and bacon bits. Website: pizzahut.co.uk.

Subway subs can be ordered as a salad (request no croutons), including the Chicken and Bacon, Subway Melt, Steak and Cheese, and Spicy Italian. Also okay are the salad with vinaigrette dressing. Website: subway.co.uk.

CASUAL DINING, YOUR WAY

When you're not in the mood for fast food but don't want to make a big dent in your wallet, there's another kind of chain restaurant you can patronise. Casual dining restaurants such as Nandos, T.G.I. Friday's and Frankie & Benny's also offer more choices and opportunities to "have it your way" in terms of sauces, pickles, cheeses, and add-ons for burgers, chicken, steaks, salads, and other main courses. However, you'll still have to be alert for the same minefield of monster portions, sauces and dressings full of sugar, and a bevy of battered and breaded dishes. Most of these eateries have lengthy menus, and among the sea of high-carb options you can find some Atkins-friendly items. You may want to ask that half the meal be put in a doggy bag before you begin, so you can have it for lunch the next day. Let's visit a few of the more popular casual dining chains.

Barburrito offers the option of a burrito bowl served over a bed of chopped romaine instead of in a tortilla or without the rice and beans. Or put together a meal from several sides, such as guacamole; salsa; mixed grilled peppers, chillies, and onion; and grilled chicken or steak. Website: barburrito.co.uk.

T.G.I. Friday's offer some good options. Try the Steak, ribs, shrimp, salmon fillet or chicken without sauce. Website: tgifridays.co.uk.

Frankie & Benny's take Italian cuisine beyond pasta and breaded main courses. Try mixed grill without fries, sirloin or rib-eye with a side salad or steak or salmon citrus salad. Website: Frankieandbennys.com.

Nandos offer a selection of chicken dishes such as Butterfly Chicken, Chicken Wings or Chicken Leg (ask for sauce on the side). Other choices include Avocado and Green Bean Salad, Mediterranean Salad or Mixed Leaf Salad.

NAVIGATING DIFFICULT SITUATIONS

Some places pose more of a challenge to Atkins followers than others. And sometimes the best alternative is still not ideal, but hey, we live in the real world. So let's check out what your best choices are at pizza places, coffee shops, vending machines, convenience stores, and more.

- *A pizza place.* Yes, you can resort to the old (and messy) trick of scraping the toppings off the pizza crust, but instead, order an antipasto plate or a salad topped with grilled chicken. If pizza is the only thing on the menu, opt for a thin-crust version, preferably made with wholegrain flour.
- *A coffee shop.* Whether it's Starbucks or a local joint (or even a coffee cart), order hot or iced coffee, black or with cream, rather than any of the sugar-laden concoctions. Instead of cappuccino, order caffè breve, made with espresso and single cream (instead of milk), a mocha breve, or an iced breve.

- *Vending machines.* Even offerings promoted as "healthy" are made with sugar and white flour. Opt for a bag of peanuts, pumpkin seeds, or other nuts or seeds, or have some sugar-free jerky. Although more machines now offer light meals to heat up in the microwave, they're usually based on noodles or rice, so give them a miss.
- *Petrol stations.* The choices can be pretty slim here, but possibilities include string cheese, sugar-free jerky, peanut butter, fresh fruit, a small container of plain yoghurt made with whole milk, nuts or seeds, and popcorn.

MOBILE FOOD

No time to sit down when your lunch hour is spent running errands or hitting the gym? Food carts to the rescue, and nowadays they're selling not just hot dogs and pizza, but also a host of other ethnic specialities. As food suitable for a quick bite or a meal on the run, however, most rely on a tortilla, roll, waffle, empanada, or pizza crust to contain the other ingredients. Nonetheless, you may be able to deconstruct street food to make it Atkins-friendly. Ask if you can have it on a plate instead, but don't be surprised if the vendor can't do that. If you're heading back to your workplace, when you get there simply remove the bun, pitta, rice, or other high-carb ingredient. Among the United Nations of possibilities, here are just a few:

- *American classics.* BBQ carts offer a variety of smoked ribs, chicken parts, pork loin, sausages.
- *Argentinean.* This cuisine is big on beef, but you're likely to find it stuffed into an empanada with onions, peppers, and potatoes.
- *Thai/Southeast Asian* Lemongrass-skewered chicken, pork stew with hard-boiled eggs, and grilled ribs are all typical dishes, usually served on rice.
- *Caribbean.* Usually served in a flatbread called a roti or over rice, curries are big in this cuisine; they are often served with a salad.
- *Greek or Middle Eastern.* Have kebabs, a lamb or chicken skewer, or falafel with lettuce, tomato, hummus, and cucumbers.
- *Korean.* Rice or noodles turn up in almost every dish. Simply eat the rest and leave them. Better yet, try a bento box of grilled marinated chicken and steamed vegetables. The street dish of

Korea, bi bim bop, is rice topped with sautéed seasoned vegetables, your choice of meat, and a fried egg.

You can eat Atkins-style in almost any restaurant if you know what to order. Some cuisines, such as Greek or Korean, are highly compatible with a low-carb lifestyle. Mexican and Chinese are a bit more difficult to navigate. However, in almost every case, there are Atkins-appropriate choices.

DINING OUT, ITALIAN STYLE

Italian food is a lot more than the pizza and pasta with red sauce that hail from southern Italy. Northern Italian food features rich butter and cream sauces, and the signature element in Florentine dishes is spinach. There are three basic secrets to enjoying the food at an Italian restaurant while complying with Atkins:

- Avoid the usual sides of spaghetti, polenta, or risotto.
- Ask for a bowl of olives as a starter in lieu of garlic bread.
- Ask whether dishes such as veal marsala or veal Florentine are breaded. Some chefs bread them; others don't.

Here are other ways to keep the carbs down:

HAVE THIS	INSTEAD OF THAT
Seafood salad	Battered and fried calamari
Mixed grilled vegetables or portobello mushrooms	Fried mozzarella sticks
Salad of rocket, fennel, and shaved Parmesan	Garlic bread
Antipasto platter	Stuffed clams
Endive or stracciatella soup	Fettuccini carbonara
Roasted or grilled seafood	Linguini with clam sauce
Grilled chicken breast or pork loin	Any risotto dish
Veal piccata or scaloppini	Veal or aubergine Parmesan

DINING OUT, GREEK STYLE

Greek food is based on olives, olive oil, lemons, aubergines, courgettes, spinach, fennel, vine leaves, yoghurt, garlic, mint, dill, rosemary, and tahini (ground sesame seeds). Whether at a Greek diner or an elegant restaurant, fresh fish is always a good choice. The predominant meat is lamb, but beef also appears on the menu. Request another vegetable instead of rice or flatbread. Greek salads are full of good things, including feta cheese, olives, tomatoes, and fresh basil. Steer clear of filo (phyllo), paper-thin sheets of pastry dough used in the pastry baklava as well as in savoury dishes such as spanakopita (a spinach pie). To keep the carbs down:

HAVE THIS	INSTEAD OF THAT
Tzatziki (yoghurt, cucumber, and garlic dip) spread)	Skordalia (thick potato-garlic
Avgolemono (chicken soup with egg and lemon)	Spanakopita or tyropita
Fresh vegetables and taramosalata (creamy fish roe spread)	Dolmades (stuffed vine leaves)
Braised lamb shanks	Pastitsio with pasta
Chicken grilled with lemon, garlic, and herbs	Chicken pilaf
Grilled prawns, octopus, or swordfish	Fried calamari
Cheese plate	Baklava

DINING OUT, MIDDLE EASTERN STYLE

Garlic, onions, cardamom, coriander, sesame, cumin, thyme, marjoram, and sumac are the predominant seasonings used with lamb and other meats. Many dishes, such as shish kebab and baklava, are also found in Greek cuisine. Baba ganoush, similar to hummus, is made of roasted aubergine mashed and mixed with garlic and tahini. Traditionally, baba ganoush is eaten with flatbread, but celery sticks or red pepper chunks make fine substitutes. More ways to keep the carbs down:

HAVE THIS	INSTEAD OF THAT
Loubieh (green beans with tomatoes)	Tabbouleh (bulgur salad)
Aubergine with garlic, tomatoes, and peppers	Fattoush (bread, cucumber, and tomato salad)
Lamb shish kebab	Kibbe (ground lamb and bulgur meatball meat)
Kofta (skewered and grilled lamb mince and onion meatballs)	Falafel (deep-fried chickpea balls)
Shish taouk (skewered and marinated chicken pieces grilled over charcoal)	B'steeya (Moroccan chicken pie with almonds)

DINING OUT, MEXICAN STYLE

Genuine Mexican cuisine is far more subtle and varied than the Tex-Mex, New Mexican style, and Cal-Mex variations that usually pass for Mexican cuisine in the United States and UK. Garlic, chillies, coriander, and cumin are common denominators. Fortunately, tortillas, beans, and rice are just the tip of the culinary iceberg. For starters, you can't go wrong with guacamole and salsa made without added sugar. If you're a fan of enchiladas verdes, tortillas filled with spiced chicken and covered with a tangy green sauce of tomatillos and coriander, just ask for the chicken filling minus the tortillas and topped with the sauce. Beef, chicken, or prawn fajitas are seared in a frying pan with sliced onions and peppers. Just pass on the tortillas, yellow rice, and refried beans. For other ways to keep the carbs down:

HAVE THIS	INSTEAD OF THAT
Jicama sticks	Tortilla chips
Grilled chicken wings	Stuffed jalapeño peppers or chillies rellenos
Jicama salad	Nachos
Sopa de albondigas (meatball and vegetable soup)	Quesadillas
Grilled fish (pescado)	Taco, tamale, or enchilada platter
Pollo asado (grilled chicken)	Chimichangas or flautas

Camarones al ajillo (prawns in garlic sauce)	Prawn enchiladas
Chicken or turkey mole (a complex sauce made with ground cocoa beans)	Chicken tortillas

DINING OUT, FRENCH STYLE

Choose carefully and make a few modifications, and there are plenty of Atkins-friendly dishes in French cuisine. You'll find fish, herbs, and olives in dishes that hail from Provence; butter and apples in those from Normandy; stews simmered in wine from Burgundy and Bordeaux; and sausages and beer in Alsatian specialities. Hollandaise and many other classic French sauces are based on butter or olive oil and thickened with egg yolks rather than flour. Other tips to curb the carbs: order French onion soup with Gruyère cheese, but without the toasted bread, and push the potatoes in coq au vin to the side of your plate.

HAVE THIS	INSTEAD OF THAT
Frisée salad with bacon and a poached egg	Alsatian tart (bacon, onion, and egg pie)
Coquilles St Jacques (scallops in cream sauce topped with cheese)	Lobster in puff pastry
Mussels in white wine sauce or bouillabaisse (fish stew)	Vichyssoise (cream of leek and potato soup)
Coq au vin	Duck à l'orange or aux cerises
Entrecôte or tournedos Bordelaise (steak in shallot and red wine sauce)	Croque monsieur (fried ham and cheese sandwich)
Veal Marengo	Veal Prince Orloff
Cheese plate	Crêpes Suzette

DINING OUT, INDIAN STYLE

Indian food comprises a varied collection of regional cuisines. Although many dishes rely on rice and other grains, you'll also find lamb, duck, chicken, and even goat on the menu. The typical Indian menu offers many choices that provide a good balance of protein and fibre-rich vegetables. Just stay away from breads, rice, and other starchy dishes. Tandoori dishes are among the most popular Indian offerings, followed by curries. You'll also find grilled kebabs and dals, which are lentil, chickpea, or bean dishes. Try raita, which is yoghurt mixed with minced cucumber and mint, to ease the heat of some of the hotter curries. To cut the carbs:

HAVE THIS	INSTEAD OF THAT
Shahi paneer (cheese in a creamy curried tomato sauce)	Vegetable samosas (savoury pastries)
Roasted aubergine with onions and spices	Pakora (fritters)
Chicken shorba	Mulligatawny soup
Tandoori chicken or other meat	Vindaloo (contains potatoes)
Korma (meat in a cream sauce)	Biryani (a rice dish)
Chicken, fish, or meat curry	Dal
Chicken, lamb, or prawn kebabs	Chicken or lamb saag

DINING OUT, CHINESE STYLE

Rice and noodles are the staples of the four major regional cuisines: Cantonese, Szechuan, Hunan, and Shandong. Most dishes use meat or fish as an addition rather than the main ingredient and rely on a sauce – generally thickened with cornflour. If possible, request that any dish be prepared with the sauce on the side. Mu shu duck, for example, is usually dusted with almond flour, fried, and served with a dark brown sauce. The sauce is sweetened, but the duck itself is delicious without it. Avoid any sweet-and-sour and breaded or battered dishes as well as noodle dishes. A small portion of brown rice is fine, if your carb tolerance allows. Have Peking duck and mu shu pork but skip the pancakes and plum sauce. To avoid empty carbs:

HAVE THIS	INSTEAD OF THAT
Clear egg drop soup (without cornflour)	Fried wontons
Hot-and-sour soup	Egg roll
Sizzling prawn platter	Prawn fried rice
Steamed or stir-fried tofu with vegetables	Deep-fried tofu dish
Beef with Chinese mushrooms	Any noodle-based dish
Stir-fried pork with garlic sauce	Sweet-and-sour pork
Peking duck	General Tso's chicken

DINING OUT, JAPANESE STYLE

White rice is a staple of this cuisine, but you can still enjoy Japanese food without it. Sauces and seasonings include shoyu, or Japanese soya sauce; mirin, sweet rice wine that usually contains added sugar; dashi, stock made from dried fish (bonito) flakes; ponzu, a dipping sauce made from shoyu, rice wine vinegar, dashi, and seaweed; wasabi, an extremely hot Japanese horseradish; pickled ginger; miso, a paste made from fermented soybeans; and sesame seeds and toasted sesame oil. A variety of vegetables are usually grilled or blanched briefly. Try burdock (a relative of the artichoke), daikon, lotus root, and Japanese aubergine. Also sample the pickled vegetables, including seaweed, which are most often served as a snack or appetiser. Oshinko means "pickle" in Japanese, but these are unlike any gherkins you've ever tried. For a fun-to-eat, satisfying main course, try shabu-shabu, thin slices of beef and vegetables that you cook at the table in stock – it's the Japanese version of fondue. To cut the carbs:

HAVE THIS	INSTEAD OF THAT
Sashimi	Sushi
Oshinko, edamame, steamed vegetables or grilled aubergine	Gyoza (fried vegetable dumplings)
Shabu-shabu	Sukiyaki
Grilled fish or prawns with soya or ginger sauce	Prawn tempura
Grilled squid	Seafood noodle dishes
Negamaki (spring onions wrapped in thin-sliced beef)	Beef teriyaki (contains added sugar)

DINING OUT, THAI STYLE

Pad thai, the national dish, is based on noodles with prawns, spring onions, eggs, dried tofu, bean sprouts, and chopped peanuts. But the flavours and combinations that make Thai food distinctive, including coconut milk, lemongrass, tamarind, coriander, turmeric, cumin, chillies, lime juice, and lime leaves, can be found in many other dishes. For example, nua yang nam tok is made with sliced steak marinated in lime juice and mixed with chillies, onion, tomato, cucumber, coriander leaves, and lettuce. The same flavours are applied to sliced squid in yum pla muk. Try tom yum goong, a prawn soup with straw mushrooms, seasoned with lime juice, lemongrass, and hot peppers; or gai tom kha, made with chicken slices in coconut milk. In general, it's best to stick to dishes that are quickly sautéed with vegetables and aromatic Thai herbs. To keep a lid on carbs:

HAVE THIS	INSTEAD OF THAT
Tom yum goong	Dumplings or spring rolls
Sautéed prawns with basil, chilli, and onion	Pad thai
Sautéed scallops with mushrooms, courgettes and chilli paste	Curried scallops with potatoes
Sautéed prawns with prawn paste and green beans sauce	Sautéed prawns with black bean
Sautéed mixed vegetables	Fried rice

DINING OUT, KOREAN STYLE

Fish and shellfish, usually grilled or stewed in a sauce, make up a large part of the typical Korean diet. Pork, beef, and chicken are often marinated and grilled. Some dishes, such as kalbi tang, a marinated beef rib stew, are served with rice; others come with noodles. Korea is also known for its barbecue (bulgogi) of thin slices of a premium cut of beef. A Korean restaurant may also offer barbecued chicken and pork, and perhaps fish and squid bulgogi, but skip the sauce, which is likely sweetened with sugar. Kimchi, an assortment of fermented vegetables seasoned with hot chillies, salt, garlic, onions, ginger, and oyster or fish sauce, is one of the best-known Korean specialities. To keep carbs under control:

HAVE THIS	INSTEAD OF THAT
Cold tofu	Pa jon (spring onion pancake)
Twoenjangguk (soup of fermented soybean paste and baby clams)	Korean dumplings
Shinsollo (hotpot of meat or fish, vegetables and tofu)	Any rice dish
Any barbecued dish	Any rice or noodle dish

BE ON YOUR *GUEST* BEHAVIOUR

Dining at a friend or relative's house should be an enjoyable occasion. But you may fear that your host or hostess will be offended if you don't eat everything, exclaim how fabulous it is, and ask for seconds. What to do if you know that some of the dishes aren't going to pass muster carb-wise? To a large degree, it depends on the circumstances.

- *The meal is buffet style.* You're in luck. Simply pick the items you can eat and pass on the others. If people are sitting all over the house or garden, it's unlikely your host will notice what each guest selects.
- *The invitation says potluck.* Bring a low-carb dish and share it. Also have suitable foods prepared by others, such as salad or vegetables.
- *It's a sit-down affair.* Your host and/or hostess are in charge, and your relationship with them is more important than avoiding a few grams of added sugar or a spoonful of potatoes au gratin. That doesn't mean that you're not within your rights to ask for sauce on the side or for a small portion of a high-carb dish. When it comes to pudding, ask for a small piece, take a bite, and leave the rest on the plate.

Many people have food allergies or dietary preferences. If your host had to accommodate the personal food issues of every guest, he or she might never get a meal on the table! However, if you're asked before the event whether there's anything you don't eat, you certainly can say that you're slimming down and are staying away from puddings and starches. Immediately add that by no means should that influence the menu. Instead, just eat the main dish and vegetables.

EATING ON THE ROAD

When you're on your own turf, it's always easier to stick to your usual routine. If you travel for business or pleasure, your usual patterns may be disrupted by time-zone changes, a schedule you don't control, or countless other factors. Before you leave the house:

- If you have to be up at dawn, grab an Atkins bar or prepare a low-carb breakfast for yourself the night before. Have it before you go or take it with you. Don't leave home empty-handed or on an empty stomach.
- Know where to find acceptable snacks or meals so that if you can't bring something with you, at least you know the location of a convenience store or fast-food place with low-carb options along the way.
- One item will do as a snack, but if you're putting together a meal, you'll need to include several items. Pack each item in a separate resealable bag in an insulated carrier.
- Bring suitable foods such as the ones listed as snacks appropriate for the various phases (see pages 76–7, 112–113, and 138–143) to keep you satisfied and able to resist temptation.

If you're on holiday and sightseeing or engaging in activities such as hiking, swimming, or skiing, chances are you're getting plenty of exercise. But if you're spending most of your waking hours in a conference room or driving from one appointment to another, you'll probably want to find a way to get some physical activity. Many hotels have a fitness centre or gym; if not, you can always bring your walking shoes and get out and explore the surroundings.

ON THE WING

Your commitment to eating the Atkins way needn't be disrupted en route if you follow these suggestions for a smooth flight.

- Atkins bars are great portable snacks – just don't try to carry a shake on a plane! (Like all beverages, it can't go through security.)
- Bring suitable food from home packed in a way that will pass muster at security.
- Alternatively, after security clearance, visit a salad bar. Pile up the greens and top them with slices of chicken or another protein source to take with you on the plane. Also purchase bottled water, soda water, unsweetened tea, coffee, or herbal tea so that you can stay hydrated in the air.
- Go to the website for the carrier you're flying on and check out the meal options to ensure that something suitable is available. Most airlines have a main-dish salad that will serve.
- Bring small bags of nuts or seeds with you to munch on.

LOW-CARB ROOM SERVICE

Staying in a hotel can be a nice break from your usual responsibilities. No need to make dinner – or the bed! But the room's refrigerator is likely full of the same high-carb foods you've banished from your own kitchen: biscuits, sweets, crackers, and crisps. If you fear that you'll be tempted, decline the key to the fridge or return it to the front desk. Room service is wonderfully convenient, but it too poses some challenges:

- Specify what you don't want – no toast, bread, or jam, for example – as well as what you do want.
- Have the server immediately remove anything you don't want tempting you if it arrives despite your instructions.
- As soon as you've eaten, put the tray outside the door.

Whether you're eating out, travelling, or grabbing a meal during your lunch break, with this wealth of information you'll undoubtedly feel more in control of your meals away from home. In the next chapter, I hope to lure you back into your own kitchen to try out some delicious quick and easy Atkins recipes, all of which are acceptable from day one on Atkins.

PART IV

RECIPES

RECIPE INDEX

BREAKFAST

LUNCH OR DINNER DISHES

SAUCES

MAIN DISH SALADS

SOUPS, CHOWDERS, AND CHILLI

SNACKS

DESSERTS

COOK'S NOTES

Most of the ingredients found in the following recipes are available in your supermarket. Sources for a few less familiar ingredients are provided.

Several of the recipes call for coconut-flax flour blend. To make, mix equal parts coconut flour with ground flax seed and refrigerate in an airtight container. Both ingredients can be found in most supermarkets in the baking aisle or gluten-free section, as well as at health food shops. If you opt to use only ground flax seed in baking, the texture will not be as cake-like and some people find the taste bitter. For best results, flax seed should be finely ground in a coffee grinder or mini food processor; most pre-ground brands are chunky. The coconut-flax flour blend also dials down the carbs but preserves a soft cake-like texture. Some recipes call for tamari, which contains no wheat, rather than soya sauce, which does. However, if you have no tamari on hand, feel free to substitute soya sauce.

Some recipes call for both cooking spray (use the rapeseed oil or olive oil kind) and oil or butter. Use the cooking spray first to lubricate the pan, which enables the oil or butter to spread more evenly, reducing the risk of items such as crêpes sticking to the pan.

Nutrition figures per serving have been rounded off to the nearest whole gram. Also provided is the number of grams of foundation vegetables in each serving. We used Stevia when calculating nutrition figures; other acceptable sweeteners include sucralose, saccharin, xylitol, and maltitol, as well as a new entry, lo han guao, made from an extract of monk fruit.

All recipes are acceptable for Phases 1 to 4. If a variation is suitable only for later phases, that is indicated. Note that the inclusion of nuts and seeds in Phase 1 is acceptable in both Atkins products and recipes if the Net Carb count is appropriate for this phase, because nuts and seeds do not provoke a blood-sugar response.

Recipes are coded as follows:

7 No more than seven ingredients (plus salt and pepper)

Total prep time of 20 minutes or less

Make-ahead recipes that can be refrigerated or frozen

SC Can be made in a slow cooker

Active Time: Preparation time

Total Time: Total time for preparation and cooking

BREAKFASTS

Courgette-Pumpkin Spice Pancakes

Courgette and pumpkin pancakes make great puddings and breakfast fare. Top with sugar-free breakfast syrup and/or a dollop of mascarpone. Allow leftover pancakes to cool completely, wrap individually in cling film, and freeze for up to 3 months. Reheat in a toaster oven for 10 minutes or in a preheated 150°C (300°F) oven for 15 minutes. Be sure to use plain tinned pumpkin, not pumpkin pie filling, which is full of sugar.

Makes: 4 servings (12 pancakes)
Active Time: 10 minutes
Total Time: 40 minutes

4 large eggs, separated
175 g (6 oz) courgette, grated
115 g (4 oz) tinned pumpkin
125 ml (4 fl oz) plain unsweetened soya milk
1 teaspoon acceptable sweetener
40 g (1½ oz) coconut-flax flour blend
2 tablespoons plain unsweetened protein powder
¼ teaspoon salt
½ teaspoon baking powder
½ teaspoon pumpkin pie spice mix
Rapeseed oil or olive oil cooking spray
4 teaspoons rapeseed oil

1. Using an electric mixer on high speed, whisk the egg whites and a small pinch of salt in a large bowl until stiff peaks form. Set aside.
2. Place the egg yolks, courgettes, pumpkin, soya milk, and sweetener in another large bowl and mix well.
3. Combine the coconut-flax flour blend, protein powder, salt, baking powder, and pumpkin pie spice in a small bowl. (Or mix on a sheet of baking parchment to avoid having to wash another bowl.)
4. Sprinkle the dry ingredients over the egg yolk mixture and a large spoonful of the beaten egg whites. Fold until combined. Fold in the remaining egg whites until the mixture is light and fluffy.

5. Coat a large frying pan or griddle with cooking spray and place it over medium heat. Add 1 teaspoon oil. Using 6 tablespoons of the batter, drop 3 mounds of batter into the pan, and smooth out with the back of a spoon (each pancake will be 2 tablespoons of batter). Cook 2–3 minutes, until edges are slightly browned. Flip and cook 2–3 minutes more, until firm in the middle. Transfer to a warmed plate and repeat three times with remaining pancake batter, using 1 teaspoon rapeseed oil each time. Serve immediately.

PER SERVING: Net Carbs: 4 grams; Fibre: 4 grams; Protein: 14 grams; Fat: 13 grams; Calories: 198; Foundation Vegetables Net Carbs: 2 grams

VARIATIONS

- In place of the coconut-flax flour blend, use 40 g (1½ oz) finely ground flaxseed.
- Swap yellow summer squash for the courgette.
- Phases 3 and 4: Substitute grated apple – no need to peel it – for courgette.

Eggs Parmesan

To make this one-dish meal an equally tasty lunch or light dinner, add sausages or bacon. Serve with your favourite hot sauce, if you wish.

Makes: 4 servings
Active Time: 10 minutes
Total Time: 15 minutes

1 tablespoon virgin olive oil
525 g (1 lb 2 oz) broccoli, roughly chopped
100 g (3½ oz) tomato sauce, bottled or tinned
4 large eggs
55 g (2 oz) grated mozzarella
100 g (3½ oz) finely grated Parmesan cheese
Salt and freshly ground black pepper

1. Heat a large frying pan over high heat and add the oil. Add the broccoli and cook 2–3 minutes, stirring frequently, until it begins to soften.

218

2. Turn the heat to low and spoon the tomato sauce over the broccoli. Break the eggs over the sauce, spacing them 10 cm (4 in) apart. Sprinkle with mozzarella and then Parmesan.
3. Cover and cook 4 to 5 minutes, until the cheese has melted and the whites of the eggs are cooked through but the yolks are still slightly runny.
4. Using a spatula, spoon out four portions, each with an egg in the middle, into bowls. Sprinkle with salt and pepper and serve immediately.

PER SERVING: Net Carbs: 4 grams; Fibre: 2 grams; Protein: 19 grams; Fat: 17 grams; Calories: 252; Foundation Vegetables Net Carbs: 2 grams

VARIATIONS

- Substitute cauliflower for broccoli.
- In Phase 2 and beyond, slide each portion into low-carb pitta.

Chocolate Waffles

The whole family will enjoy these sweet, tender waffles. Top each waffle with a dollop of whipping cream if you wish. Be sure to use unsweetened cocoa, not hot chocolate mix.

Makes: 4 (1-waffle) servings
Active Time: 10 minutes
Total Time: 30 minutes

4 large eggs, separated
¼ teaspoon salt
175 ml (6 fl oz) plain unsweetened soya milk
125 g (4½ oz) mascarpone
2 tablespoons melted butter, cooled
1 teaspoon acceptable sweetener
1 teaspoon vanilla extract
40 g (1½ oz) coconut-flax flour blend
2 tablespoons unsweetened protein powder
2 tablespoons unsweetened cocoa powder
½ teaspoon baking powder
Rapeseed oil or olive oil cooking spray

1. Using an electric mixer on high speed, whisk the egg whites and salt in a large bowl until stiff peaks form. Set aside.
2. In a second bowl, whisk egg yolks, soya milk, mascarpone, butter, sweetener, and vanilla. Add the coconut-flax flour blend, protein powder, cocoa powder, and baking powder and stir to combine.
3. Add a large spoonful of egg whites to the egg yolk mixture. Using a rubber spatula, fold in the egg whites and all of the flour until just combined, about 8 turns, forming a sticky mass. Fold in another large spoonful of egg whites until the mixture becomes lighter, an additional 4–5 turns. Finally, fold in the remaining egg whites. There will be small lumps but don't overmix.
4. Heat a waffle iron according to the manufacturer's instructions and mist with cooking spray. Add a quarter of the batter and spread it evenly with the back of a spoon. Cover and cook 2–3 minutes or until the waffle is firm and light brown. Repeat with remaining batter and serve immediately. Or cool to room temperature, double-wrap in cling film, and freeze.

PER SERVING: Net Carbs: 3 grams; Fibre: 4 grams; Protein: 16 grams; Fat: 26 grams; Calories: 326; Foundation Vegetables Net Carbs: 0 grams

VARIATIONS

- In place of the coconut-flax flour blend, use 40 g (1½ oz) finely ground flaxseed.
- In Phase 2, top with fresh or frozen raspberries or strawberries.

Breakfast Casserole ◐ ▤

Ideal for the beginner cook, this dish can be made ahead and reheated. If you're unaccustomed to cooking with leafy greens such as kale, this rich, cheesy recipe is a great way to start. You can also serve it for lunch or dinner.

Makes: 4 servings
Active Time: 10 minutes
Total Time: 35 minutes

1 tablespoon virgin olive oil
2 Italian sausages, chopped
85 g (3 oz) chopped red onion
225 g (8 oz) button or cremini mushrooms, chopped
225 g (8 oz) sliced packed kale (stems and ribs removed)
8 large eggs, lightly beaten
100 g (3½ oz) grated Cheddar cheese
1 teaspoon baking powder
Salt and freshly ground black pepper

1. Preheat oven to 200°C (400°F). Warm a large frying pan over medium heat. Add the olive oil, sausage, and onion. Cook 3–4 minutes, breaking up the sausage with the back of a wooden spoon as it browns. Add the mushrooms and cook 1 minute more, until they soften. Add the kale and set aside to cool for 5 minutes.
2. Meanwhile, in a large bowl, whisk together the eggs, cheese, and baking powder. Add the sausage mixture and transfer to a 20-cm (8-in) square baking dish lined with aluminium foil.
3. Bake uncovered 20–25 minutes, until the eggs puff up and the casserole is firm in the centre. Cool 5 minutes, then slice into 4 even wedges. Season with salt and pepper and serve immediately.

PER SERVING: Net Carbs: 7 grams; Fibre: 1 gram; Protein: 26 grams; Fat: 32 grams; Calories: 414; Foundation Vegetables Net Carbs: 5 grams

VARIATIONS

- Use crumbled cooked bacon, cubed ham, cooked turkey cubes, or other leftovers in place of sausage.
- Substitute spinach or rocket for kale.

Breakfast Sandwich 🌓 ▤

There's a surprise ingredient in this savoury homemade "flatbread" that makes this sandwich a protein all-star: minced chicken! If you don't have any leftover chicken, use grilled or roasted skinless chicken from the deli department. Mince the chicken in the food processor.

Makes: 2 servings
Active Time: 10 minutes
Total Time: 25 minutes

1 large egg
60 g (2¼ oz) minced cooked chicken
50 g (1¾ oz) finely grated Parmesan cheese
2 tablespoons ground flaxseed
½ teaspoon Italian seasoning (optional)
Olive oil or rapeseed oil cooking spray
2 rashers cooked bacon, roughly chopped
2 slices Cheddar cheese
    (approx. 18 g/¾ oz each)
Salt and freshly ground black pepper

1. Preheat the oven to 230°C (450°F). To make the flatbread, first whisk the egg in a large bowl. Add the minced chicken, Parmesan, flaxseed, and Italian seasoning, if using, and mix until it forms a heavy dough.
2. Coat a 20-cm (8-in) square baking dish with cooking spray. Add the dough and press it into the pan using the back of a fork, forming an even layer. The surface of the dough will have ridges.
3. Bake 8–10 minutes, until firm. Cut the flatbread into 4 even squares.
4. Layer two squares of the flatbread with bacon and top each with a slice of Cheddar cheese and then another flatbread square. Press

down firmly and bake an additional 3–4 minutes, until the cheese melts.

5. Season with salt and pepper and serve immediately. Or wrap in greaseproof paper to go. Reheat in a 200°C (400°F) oven for 10 minutes.

PER SERVING: Net Carbs: 1 gram; Fibre: 1 gram; Protein: 23 grams; Fat: 17 grams; Calories: 245; Foundation Vegetables Net Carbs: 0 grams

VARIATIONS

- Instead of bacon, use a cooked sausage, cut into 8 thin slices.
- Add leftover vegetables such as sautéed spinach and/or mushrooms.
- Make crackers with the flatbread dough by following steps 1–3. Remove from the pan and cool completely on a plate before wrapping in cling film and refrigerating for up to 4 days, or freeze for up to 3 months in a resealable bag.

LUNCH OR DINNER DISHES

Deep-Dish Sausage and Cauliflower Pizza ◑ ▤

If you devour this delicious pizza the minute it comes out of the oven, you'll need a knife and fork. Let it cool for 10 minutes, though, and the crust will firm up, so you can use your fingers. It also keeps nicely in the refrigerator for up to 3 days, wrapped in greaseproof paper and cling film. Use frozen cauliflower, if you wish.

Makes: 4 servings
Active Time: 10 minutes
Total Time: 25 minutes

Rapeseed oil or olive oil cooking spray
1 large egg
325 g (11½ oz) cooked and roughly chopped cauliflower*
150 g (5½ oz) grated mozzarella (full fat)
115 g (4 oz) bottled no-sugar-added tomato sauce
3 cooked sausages, thinly sliced
15 g (½ oz) spinach, finely chopped
Salt and freshly ground black pepper

1. Preheat the oven to 230°C (450°F). Coat a 20-cm (8-in) square baking dish with cooking spray.
2. Place the egg in a large bowl and whisk by hand until foamy. Add cauliflower and 100 g (3½ oz) mozzarella; stir well. Press the cauliflower mixture evenly into the baking dish.
3. Bake 10–12 minutes, until the crust is golden and firm. Remove from the oven and spread the tomato sauce over the crust, then sprinkle with sausage, spinach, and the remaining mozzarella. Season with salt and pepper.
4. Return the pizza to the oven and bake 2 more minutes, just until the cheese melts. Slice into 4 equal pieces and serve immediately.

*To roughly chop the cauliflower, cut into florets and steam 5–6 minutes over boiling water until fork tender. You'll need 400g (14 oz) florets to make 325 g (11½ oz) of roughly chopped cauliflower. Use a potato masher or fork, or transfer to a food processor in batches and blitz to roughly chop. Cool completely before using in recipes. Roughly chopped cauliflower keeps for 4 days in the refrigerator in an airtight container. Or freeze for up to 3 months.

PER SERVING: Net Carbs: 4 grams; Fibre: 2 grams; Protein: 18 grams; Fat: 26 grams; Calories: 331; Foundation Vegetables Net Carbs: 3 grams

VARIATIONS

• Top pizza with 50 g (1¾ oz) sliced mushrooms, drained marinated artichokes, roasted red peppers, or chopped olives.

Cheesy Chicken and Green Bean Sauté ◑ ⊟

If your family loves creamy casseroles but doesn't want to wait 45 minutes, this is your dish. Cheesy and rich, but quick and easy to make, this is comfort food at its best! To get dinner on the table faster, do the prep work the night before or earlier in the day – cut up the chicken, beans, mushrooms, and onions, and grate the cheese. Then store in sealed containers in the refrigerator until you're ready to prepare.

Makes: 4 servings
Active Time: 10 minutes
Total Time: 20 minutes

675 g (1 lb 8 oz) uncooked chicken breast, cut into 5-cm (2-in) cubes
½ teaspoon paprika
½ teaspoon garlic powder
2 tablespoons butter
300 g (10½ oz) green beans, cut into 2.5-cm (1-in) lengths
225 g (8 oz) mushrooms (button or cremini), thinly sliced
½ small red onion, finely chopped
½ teaspoon salt
2 tablespoons coconut-flax flour blend
125 ml (4 fl oz) soya milk or chicken stock
100 g (3½ oz) grated Cheddar cheese
¼ teaspoon freshly ground black pepper

1. Place chicken cubes on a plate, sprinkle with paprika and garlic powder, and set aside.
2. Warm a large, deep frying pan over medium heat. Add the butter, green beans, mushrooms, and onion. Sprinkle the vegetables with salt and cook 4 to 5 minutes, stirring occasionally, until the onion softens.
3. Add the chicken and the coconut-flax flour blend and cook for 1 minute, stirring to distribute the flour blend. Add the soya milk or chicken stock and cover. Reduce the heat to low and simmer for 1–2 minutes, or until the chicken is cooked through.
4. Scatter the cheese over the top of the chicken, season with pepper, and cover. Turn off the heat and leave on the hob for 1–2 minutes, until the cheese melts. Serve immediately.

PER SERVING: Net Carbs: 6 grams; Fibre: 3 grams; Protein: 46 grams; Fat: 21 grams; Calories: 405; Foundation Vegetables Net Carbs: 4 grams

VARIATIONS

- In place of the coconut-flax flour blend, use 40 g (1½ oz) finely ground flaxseed.
- Replace the green beans with broccoli.
- Top with 10 g (¼ oz) chopped fresh basil.
- Phases 2–4: Serve over Atkins Penne or Fusilli Pasta.

Asian Beef Stir-Fry ◯ ⊟

Chinese takeaway is convenient, but it can be full of hidden sugars. Instead, make this quick and easy version of a classic dish flavoured with orange zest. Pre-sliced beef strips are great time savers, as is bottled or frozen grated ginger. Like most Chinese food, leftovers can be reheated.

Makes: 4 servings
Active Time: 10 minutes
Total Time: 20 minutes

675 g (1½ lb) beef strips for stir-frying
2 teaspoons orange zest
   (or ¼ teaspoon orange extract)
1 tablespoon coconut-flax flour blend
1 tablespoon rapeseed oil
1 tablespoon sesame oil
675 g (1½ lb) broccoli
1 red pepper, seeded, thinly sliced
2 garlic cloves, finely chopped
1 tablespoon freshly grated ginger (optional)
225 ml (8 fl oz) beef stock
2 tablespoons tamari
Freshly ground black pepper

1. Place the beef strips on a plate and scatter over the orange zest and coconut-flax flour blend. Heat a large, deep frying pan or wok over high heat. Add the rapeseed oil and beef. Cook 2–3 minutes, stirring often, until the beef starts to brown. Transfer to a plate.
2. Reduce the heat to medium. Add the sesame oil, broccoli, red pepper, garlic, and ginger, if using. Cook 2–3 minutes, stirring often, until the vegetables begin to soften. Return beef to the pan along with the stock and tamari. Cook 1 minute more, until the beef is cooked through. Season with black pepper and serve immediately.

PER SERVING: Net Carbs: 6 grams; Fibre: 4 grams; Protein: 42 grams; Fat: 22 grams; Calories: 408; Foundation Vegetables Net Carbs: 5 grams

VARIATIONS

- Omit the coconut-flax flour blend, but do not use all flaxseed.
- Replace the broccoli with mangetout or sliced asparagus. Or add tinned water chestnuts or palm hearts.
- Phases 3–4: Serve over brown rice.

Slow Cooker Pork and Salsa Verde Parcels ◐ ▤ sc

With 6 servings, this recipe is ideal for planned leftovers. Instead of wrapping the pork and sauce in lettuce leaf parcels you can also ladle it over the lettuce. Make the pork filling up to 3 days ahead, cool completely, and refrigerate in an airtight container.

Makes: 6 (3-roll) servings
Active Time: 10 minutes
Total Time: 4 hours, 20 minutes

1 tablespoon rapeseed oil
900 g (2 lb) boneless pork loin end roast
½ teaspoon mild chilli powder
350 ml (12 fl oz) bottled no-sugar-added salsa verde
1 lime, zest and juice
   (or 2 tablespoons bottled lime juice)
18 butter or other soft lettuce leaves
200 g (7 oz) cherry tomatoes, chopped
100 g (3¾ oz) finely shredded red cabbage
18 coriander sprigs (optional)
Salt and freshly ground black pepper

1. Heat a large, deep frying pan over high heat. Add oil and pork and sear for 3–4 minutes, without moving, until golden brown. Sprinkle with chilli powder and turn over. Cook another 3–4 minutes, until the other side is golden brown.
2. Transfer to the dish of your slow cooker and set to high following the manufacturers' instructions. Add the salsa verde, lime zest and juice, and seasoning. Cover and cook for 4 hours on high. Remove the pork from the slow cooker and let it rest for about 5 minutes or until cool enough to handle. Shred with your fingers or two forks, then return the meat to the slow cooker. Turn off the slow cooker.
3. To serve, place about 2 tablespoons shredded meat and sauce into a lettuce leaf and top with 1 tablespoon tomatoes and 1 tablespoon cabbage. Roll up the parcel, top with a sprig of coriander, if using, and serve immediately.

PER SERVING: Net Carbs: 6 grams; Fibre: 1 gram; Protein: 32 grams; Fat: 9 grams; Calories: 250; Foundation Vegetables Net Carbs: 6 grams

VARIATIONS

- Replace the pork with an equal amount of chicken breast on the bone; decrease cooking time by an hour. Remove the bones and shred.
- Serve with a dollop of soured cream.
- Phases 2–4: Roll in a small low-carb tortilla.

Tilapia Fish Cakes on Baby Spinach

Love crab cakes but not the cost? Here's an inexpensive alternative. Tilapia takes well to seasoning and is palatable to those who aren't big fish fans. These fish cakes can be made up to 5 hours ahead. Just form and coat the cakes, then refrigerate – you can do the actual cooking when family or guests arrive. If you use frozen tilapia, defrost in the refrigerator overnight before cooking.

Makes: 4 servings
Active Time: 15 minutes
Total Time: 40 minutes

175 g (6 oz) baby spinach
3 tablespoons virgin olive oil, divided
675 g (1½ lb) fresh tilapia fillet
125 g (4½ oz) rapeseed oil mayonnaise
2 tablespoons spring onions, white and
    green parts, thinly sliced
2 tablespoons fresh parsley, chopped
2 teaspoons Dijon mustard
½ teaspoon salt
40 g (1½ oz) coconut-flax flour blend
2 tablespoons grated Parmesan cheese
1 lemon, quartered

1. Divide the spinach between four plates. Heat a large, deep frying pan over high heat and add 1 tablespoon olive oil. Reduce heat to medium and add the tilapia. Cover and cook 6–7 minutes, turning once or twice, until cooked through. Transfer to a large bowl to cool slightly.

2. Add the mayonnaise, spring onions, parsley, mustard, and salt to the bowl of tilapia. Fold all the ingredients together until the mixture comes together in a sticky mass.
3. Shape the tilapia mixture into eight 10-cm (4-in) diameter cakes. Place the coconut-flax flour blend and Parmesan on a plate or piece of greaseproof paper. Mix with your fingertips.
4. Roll the fish cakes in the Parmesan–coconut-flax mixture and place on another piece of greaseproof paper.
5. Wipe the frying pan clean and add the remaining 2 tablespoons oil. Add the fish cakes and cook 3–4 minutes. Turn and cook an additional 4 minutes. You may have to cook these in two batches. Place 2 fish cakes on to each plate beside the spinach and serve immediately with lemon wedges on the side.

PER SERVING: Net Carbs: 4 grams; Fibre: 5 grams; Protein: 37 grams; Fat: 38 grams; Calories: 517; Foundation Vegetables Net Carbs: 2 grams

VARIATIONS

- In place of the coconut-flax flour blend, use 40 g (1½ oz) finely ground flaxseed.
- Use salmon (including tinned salmon), cod, or haddock for the tilapia.
- Omit the baby spinach and serve over creamed spinach (see page 226).
- Serve with Lemon Tartare Sauce (page 223) instead of lemon wedges.

SAUCES

Lemon Tartare Sauce

Use this versatile sauce with chicken, fish, or pork. It also makes a tangy dip for crudités. Try it as a dressing drizzled over cooked or raw leafy greens, as well as cooked broccoli, green beans, or asparagus. Or use it instead of mayo in tuna or salmon salad.

Makes: 8 (2-tablespoon) servings
Active Time: 5 minutes
Total Time: 5 minutes

2 small gherkins, quartered
175 g (6 oz) rapeseed oil mayonnaise
25 g (1 oz) grated Parmesan cheese
1 lemon, zest and juice
    (or 2 tablespoons bottled lemon juice)
2 tablespoons double cream
½ teaspoon acceptable sweetener (optional)

1. Place the pickle in a food processor and pulse 10–15 times, until finely chopped. Add the mayonnaise, Parmesan, lemon zest and juice, cream, and sweetener, if using; process until smooth.
2. Serve immediately or refrigerate in an airtight container, for up to 1 week.

PER SERVING: Net Carbs: 1 gram; Fibre: 0 grams; Protein: 1 gram; Fat: 19 grams; Calories: 175; Foundation Vegetables Net Carbs: 0 grams

VARIATION

- Add a bit of a kick with 1 tablespoon pickled jalapeño or 1 teaspoon hot sauce.

Chipotle BBQ Sauce

Shop-bought versions of this barbecue favourite are usually packed with sugar in one form or another. This tempting, easy-to-make version uses sassy chipotle chilli to jazz up chicken, pork, or beef.

Makes: 4 (heaping 60 g/2¼ oz) servings
Active Time: 5 minutes
Total Time: 15 minutes

1 tablespoon butter
¼ small red onion, chopped
¼ teaspoon salt
225 g (8 oz) chopped tinned tomatoes
1 tablespoon tinned or bottled chipotle in adobo (see page 236), chopped
2 tablespoons red wine vinegar
1 tablespoon acceptable sweetener
1 teaspoon Dijon mustard

1. Heat a small saucepan over medium heat and add the butter. Add the onion and salt and cook 3–4 minutes, stirring occasionally, until the onion has browned. Add the chopped tomatoes, chipotle in adobo, vinegar, sweetener, and mustard. Cook 4–5 minutes, stirring occasionally, until mixture thickens.
2. Transfer to a blender or food processor and process until smooth. Serve immediately. Or store in an airtight container for a week in the refrigerator or in the freezer for up to three months.

PER SERVING: Net Carbs: 3 grams; Fibre: 1 gram; Protein: 1 gram; Fat: 3 grams; Calories: 46; Foundation Vegetables Net Carbs: 2 grams

VARIATIONS

- Use apple cider vinegar in place of red wine vinegar.
- Replace the red onion with 4 garlic cloves, thinly sliced.

Creamy Sweet Soya Sauce

This sweet but savoury sauce lends itself to multiple uses. Brush it over roast salmon, grilled chicken, or cooked prawns, or toss with sautéed kale, pak choi, or broccoli. It's great with hard-boiled eggs too. Or brush it over skewered chicken cubes or raw prawns along with vegetables such as Brussels sprouts, red and green pepper squares, and mushrooms before grilling. Finally, serve as a dip with raw vegetables.

Makes: 6 (2-tablespoon) servings
Active Time: 5 minutes
Total Time: 10 minutes

125 g (4½ oz) rapeseed oil mayonnaise
2 tablespoons tamari
3 garlic cloves, finely chopped
1 teaspoon freshly grated ginger
½ teaspoon acceptable sweetener
2 tablespoons chopped chives or spring onions (optional)

1. Place the mayonnaise, tamari, garlic, 1 tablespoon water, ginger, sweetener, and chives, if using, in a large bowl and whisk well.
2. Serve immediately or keep in the refrigerator in an airtight container for up to five days.

PER SERVING: Net Carbs: 1 gram; Fibre: 0 grams; Protein: 1 gram; Fat: 15 grams; Calories: 140; Foundation Vegetables Net Carbs: 0 grams

VARIATION

- For crispy baked chicken, coat one side of a boneless, skinless chicken breast with 1 tablespoon Creamy Sweet Soya Sauce, then press chicken into coconut-flax flour blend. Bake in a preheated oven at 180°C (350°F) uncovered and sauce side up, for 30 minutes or until done.

Parmesan-Garlic White Sauce ◔ ⊟

Step aside carbonara, there's a new sauce in town! Use this sauce thickened with coconut flour to enrich your chicken, prawns, and greens. Or wilt 125 g (4½ oz) baby spinach and top with 125 g (4½ oz) sauce for creamed spinach pronto. Sauté chicken cubes and chopped mushrooms with 1 tablespoon olive oil and top with this sauce for classic comfort food. Or top grilled or sautéed prawns with it for a creamy version of prawn scampi.

Makes: 60 g (2¼ oz) servings
Active Time: 10 minutes
Total Time: 5 minutes

1 tablespoon butter
4 garlic cloves, finely chopped
2 tablespoon coconut flour
240 ml (8 fl oz) chicken stock
100 g (3½ oz) grated Parmesan cheese
125 ml (4 fl oz) double cream
¼ teaspoon salt
¼ teaspoon freshly ground black pepper
2 tablespoons finely chopped parsley

1. Heat a saucepan over medium heat. Add the butter and garlic and cook 2–3 minutes, stirring occasionally, until the garlic is fragrant. Take care not to burn the garlic. Add the coconut flour and cook 1 minute more, until the flour coats the garlic.
2. Slowly add the stock and whisk. Bring to a simmer, and then add the Parmesan and cream. Simmer 3–4 minutes, whisking occasionally, until the mixture forms a thick sauce. Add salt, pepper, and parsley and serve immediately. It also reheats beautifully. Refrigerate in an airtight container for up to one week.

PER SERVING: Net Carbs: 2 grams; Fibre: 1 gram; Protein: 6 grams; Fat: 14 grams; Calories: 159; Foundation Vegetables Net Carbs: 0 grams

Speedy, Spicy, Chunky Tomato Sauce ◑ ⊟

This chunky sauce looks like traditional tomato sauce layered with pepperoni, but it can also be given a creamy texture. Tomato sauce isn't just for pasta. It also makes a tasty topper for green vegetables, particularly with a scattering of grated cheese.

Makes: 4 servings
Active Time: 10 minutes
Total Time: 30 minutes

1 tablespoon virgin olive oil
60 g (2¼ oz) chopped nitrate-free pepperoni
2 garlic cloves, thinly sliced
1 teaspoon red chilli flakes
½ teaspoon salt
225 g (½ lb) fresh tomatoes, chopped
1 sprig fresh basil

1. Warm a large frying pan over medium-high heat, add the olive oil, pepperoni, garlic, red chilli flakes, and salt. Cook 1–2 minutes, until the garlic is fragrant. Add the tomatoes, 125 ml (4 fl oz) water, and basil.
2. Increase the heat to high and bring to the boil. Immediately lower the heat and simmer for 18–20 minutes, until the sauce thickens. Serve immediately or refrigerate in an airtight container for up to one week.

PER SERVING: Net Carbs: 3 grams; Fibre: 1 gram; Protein: 3 grams; Fat: 7 grams; Calories: 85; Foundation Vegetables Net Carbs: 2 grams

VARIATIONS

- Use mild nitrate-free salami in place of pepperoni to reduce the heat.
- Fast, Spicy, Smooth Tomato Sauce: After Step 2, remove the basil sprig and purée the sauce in a blender. If desired, add 2 tablespoons vodka with the tomatoes and water.

MAIN DISH SALADS

Chipotle Prawn Salad

Chipotle in adobo is smoked jalapeños marinated in a garlicky tomato sauce. Look for small jars or tins in the international aisle of your supermarket. Freeze leftovers in plastic sandwich bags. For less heat, remove the seeds or reduce the amount of chipotle. You can save significantly by buying whole prawns and remove the shells and veins under cold running water before cooking. Or to save time and fuss, purchase cooked shelled prawns.

Makes: 4 servings
Active Time: 20 minutes
Total Time: 10 minutes

1 heaped tablespoon chipotle in adobo, chopped
1 lime, zest and juice
　(or 2 tablespoons bottled lime juice)
1 tablespoon extra-virgin olive oil
675 g (1½ lb) raw prawns, peeled and deveined
200 g (7 oz) finely shredded red cabbage
100 g (3½ oz) finely shredded green cabbage
20 g (¾ oz) coriander, chopped, plus extra for garnish
125 g (4½ oz) baby spinach
1 Hass avocado, peeled, seeded, and thinly sliced
2 tablespoons butter

1. Mix chipotle with the lime zest and olive oil in a large bowl. Reserve the lime juice. Add the prawns; toss to coat. In a separate bowl, toss the red and green cabbage and the coriander. Divide the spinach between four plates and top with the cabbage salad. Top each salad with ¼ avocado.
2. Heat a large frying pan over medium-high heat. Carefully add the prawn mixture and cook for 3–4 minutes, stirring often, until the prawns turn pink and are cooked through. Turn off the heat

and stir in the reserved lime juice and butter. Divide the prawn mixture between the four plates and top with the extra coriander. Serve immediately.

PER SERVING: Net Carbs: 7 grams; Fibre: 5 grams; Protein: 25 grams; Fat: 17 grams; Calories: 292; Foundation Vegetables Net Carbs: 5 grams

VARIATIONS

- Replace prawns with cubed chicken breast, adding an additional 2 minutes to cooking time. Or use leftover grilled or poached chicken breast instead, reheating for a minute or two.
- Phases 2–4: Warm low-carb tortillas, spoon prawn mixture into them, and top with the cabbage.

Grilled Chicken and Marinated Kale Salad

Kale is a mild-tasting relative of cabbage, full of vitamins A, C, and K. It's usually cooked, but is also great raw, especially after being marinated. Unlike other salads, kale doesn't go soggy or lose its flavour when stored in the refrigerator overnight, making it an excellent (and portable) leftover. Save time by using grilled chicken from a deli or salad bar.

Makes: 4 servings
Active Time: 3 hours 15 minutes
Total Time: 15 minutes

115 g (4 oz) green beans, trimmed
225 g (8 oz) kale, stems and tough ribs removed, leaves roughly torn
1 tablespoon sesame or extra-virgin olive oil
1 tablespoon red wine vinegar
½ teaspoon salt
85 g (3 oz) green or black olives, sliced
4 chicken breasts, boneless, skinless
¼ teaspoon freshly ground black pepper
1 tablespoon rapeseed oil

1. Heat 2.5 cm (1 in) of water in a medium saucepan fitted with a steamer basket over high heat. When the water boils, add the beans and steam 4–5 minutes, until fork tender. Drain and transfer to a large bowl.
2. Add the kale, sesame or olive oil, vinegar, ¼ teaspoon salt, beans, and olives to the bowl and toss gently. Cover and let rest at room temperature or in the fridge for three hours to soften the kale.
3. Heat a large frying pan over medium-high heat. Season the chicken with the remaining salt and pepper. Add the rapeseed oil and chicken to the pan. Reduce heat to medium; cook 5–6 minutes, without moving, until the chicken is well browned. Turn the chicken and cook 5–6 minutes more, until cooked through and no longer pink in the centre. Transfer to a cutting board and let rest for 5 minutes. Slice each breast into eight.
4. To serve, divide the salad among four plates, top each with eight chicken slices, and serve immediately.

PER SERVING: Net Carbs: 6 grams; Fibre: 3 grams; Protein: 39 grams; Fat: 14 grams; Calories: 313; Foundation Vegetables Net Carbs: 6 grams

VARIATIONS

- Replace the grilled chicken with leftover flank steak (see page 241).
- Substitute mangetout for green beans.
- After two weeks in Induction, top with 30 g (1 oz) chopped walnuts, divided among the plates.

Buffalo Chicken Salad

No need to worry about the carbs in bar food when you make it at home. These boneless, unbreaded chicken "fingers" are drenched in a delectable buffalo sauce that rivals what's served at the local watering hole. The minute amount of coconut flour has minimal carb impact, and the generous portion of chicken fingers turns an appetiser into a main dish.

Makes: 4 servings
Active Time: 10 minutes
Total Time: 25 minutes

240 ml (8 fl oz) beef or chicken stock
2 tablespoons Tabasco or other hot sauce
1 tablespoon tomato paste
1 tablespoon coconut flour
1 tablespoon butter
175 g (6 oz) baby spinach
85 g (3 oz) roasted red peppers, chopped
675 g (1½ lb) chicken breast,
    sliced into 24 "fingers"
½ teaspoon garlic powder
½ teaspoon mild chilli powder (optional)
1 tablespoon virgin olive oil

1. Prepare the buffalo sauce: In a small pan, stir together the stock, hot sauce, tomato paste, and coconut flour. Bring to a slow simmer and cook 5–6 minutes, until reduced slightly. Whisk in butter.
2. Toss the spinach and roasted red pepper in a large bowl. Divide the salad between four plates.
3. Season the chicken with garlic powder and chilli powder, if using.
4. Warm the olive oil in a large frying pan over medium-high heat. Add the chicken and cook 4–5 minutes, turning once, until both sides are browned. Reduce heat to low and carefully add the buffalo sauce. Transfer 6 tenders to each plate and serve immediately.

PER SERVING: Net Carbs: 5 grams; Fibre: 3 grams; Protein: 41 grams; Fat: 8 grams; Calories: 252; Foundation Vegetables Net Carbs: 4 grams

VARIATIONS

- Substitute fingers of turkey breast for chicken.
- Replace baby spinach with romaine lettuce or thinly sliced kale (stems and tough ribs removed).
- For more heat add ½ teaspoon ground cayenne pepper.

Turkey Enchilada Salad ◔

This salad uses crisp vegetables, just like the classic version, along with protein-rich turkey, but cuts the carbs.

Makes: 4 servings
Active Time: 10 minutes
Total Time: 20 minutes

450 g (1 lb) turkey steaks or escalopes
1 teaspoon mild chilli powder
½ teaspoon cumin
½ teaspoon salt
2 tablespoons rapeseed oil
1 green pepper, deseeded and chopped
115 g (4 oz) tinned no-sugar-added enchilada sauce
3 large romaine lettuces, thinly sliced
100 g (3½ oz) grated Cheddar cheese

1. Season the turkey with chilli powder, cumin, and salt. Heat a large frying pan over high heat. Add 1 tablespoon rapeseed oil and the turkey. Cook 4–5 minutes, turning once or twice, until the turkey is cooked through and no longer pink in the centre. Transfer to a warmed plate.
2. Reduce heat to medium and add the remaining tablespoon of rapeseed oil, and green pepper. Cook 2–3 minutes, stirring often, until the vegetables start to soften. Reduce heat to low and add the enchilada sauce. Stir well, scraping up any bits that stick. Turn the heat off.
3. Divide the romaine lettuce between four plates. Thinly slice the turkey steaks and divide them among the four plates. Top each plate with a quarter of the green-pepper mixture and scatter each plate with a quarter of the cheese. Serve immediately.

PER SERVING: Net Carbs: 5 grams; Fibre: 5 grams; Protein: 38 grams; Fat: 18 grams; Calories: 344; Foundation Vegetables Net Carbs: 5 grams

VARIATION

- Substitute shredded mozzarella for the Cheddar.

Crisp Lettuce Wedge with Sliced Flank Steak ◔ ☰

This steakhouse-inspired salad uses nutritious, crunchy romaine in lieu of classic iceberg lettuce. The recipe calls for 900 g (2 lb) of flank steak providing 450 g (1 lb) of leftovers for another meal, perhaps to top Marinated Kale Salad (page 237) instead of grilled chicken, or creamed spinach (see page 229). Note that the nutritional information is based on using only half the cooked flank steak.

Makes: 4 servings
Active Time: 25 minutes
Total Time: 35 minutes

2 romaine lettuces
900 g (2 lb) flank steak (in one piece)
½ teaspoon no-sugar-added steak seasoning
1 tablespoon rapeseed oil
50 ml (2 fl oz) double cream
50 ml (2 fl oz) red wine vinegar
1 tablespoon extra-virgin olive oil
1 teaspoon freshly ground black pepper
½ teaspoon garlic powder
¼ teaspoon salt
4 tablespoons crumbled blue cheese
1 red pepper, seeded, chopped
½ small red onion, sliced

1. Cut each head of romaine lettuce into four even wedges. Remove the cores, rinse under cold running water, and wrap in kitchen paper or clean tea towels. Place in the refrigerator while you prepare the steak. Season the steak with the steak seasoning.
2. Heat a large frying pan over high heat. Add the rapeseed oil along with the steak. Reduce heat to medium and cook 7–8 minutes, without moving. Turn the steak and cook 7–8 minutes more, again without moving. Transfer to a chopping board and let rest for 5 minutes.
3. Meanwhile, make the dressing: Place cream, vinegar, olive oil, black pepper, garlic powder, and salt in a medium bowl and whisk until smooth.
4. Place 2 wedges of the romaine on each of four plates. Cut the steak in half, reserving half for another recipe (see page 238 variation). Thinly slice the remaining half and divide among the four

plates. Scatter 1 tablespoon blue cheese over each salad, followed by 3 tablespoons dressing. Sprinkle with the red pepper and onion and serve immediately.

PER SERVING: Net Carbs: 4 grams; Fibre: 3 grams; Protein: 28 grams; Fat: 25 grams; Calories: 365; Foundation Vegetables Net Carbs: 3 grams

All-Season Caprese Salad with Prosciutto

Caprese salad calls for vine-ripened tomatoes, which are usually available only in late summer. This main dish version uses bottled roasted red peppers instead. You can find them in your supermarket or at any deli. Make this salad ahead, cover with cling film, and chill before transporting to your next picnic or barbecue. Serve with one of our delectable soups for a satisfying meal any time of year.

Makes: 4 servings
Active Time: 10 minutes
Total Time: 20 minutes

30 g (1 oz) parsley, stems removed
30 g (1 oz) basil, stems removed
4 tablespoons extra-virgin olive oil
4 garlic cloves, chopped
¼ teaspoon salt
8 slices prosciutto
24 spears asparagus
Rapeseed oil or olive oil cooking spray
225 g (8 oz) mozzarella
175 g (6 oz) roasted red peppers

1. Place parsley, basil, olive oil, 4 tablespoons cold water, garlic, and salt in a mini food processor or blender. Process until smooth. Set aside.
2. Cut each prosciutto slice into 3 long strips, for a total of 24. Wrap each strip around an asparagus spear; prosciutto will adhere naturally.
3. Coat a large frying pan with cooking spray. Place over high heat and add the prosciutto-wrapped asparagus. You may have to cook the asparagus in batches. Cook 5–6 minutes, turning occasionally, until the prosciutto has browned. Remove from the heat.

4. Thinly slice the mozzarella and fan it out on a platter. Top with the red peppers and prosciutto-wrapped asparagus spears and drizzle with the parsley-basil dressing. Serve immediately.

PER SERVING: Net Carbs: 7 grams; Fibre: 5 grams; Protein: 24 grams; Fat: 30 grams; Calories: 400; Foundation Vegetables Net Carbs: 5 grams

VARIATION

- Replace the roasted red peppers with two sliced vine-ripened tomatoes.
- Replace prosciutto with another 115 g (4 oz) mozzarella for a vegetarian option.

SOUPS, CHOWDERS, AND CHILLI

Cream of Romanesco Broccoli Soup

You'll need two heads of romanesco, a hybrid of cauliflower and broccoli. If you can't find romanesco, simply use one head of broccoli and one of cauliflower. You can save a bit of prep time by purchasing them as fresh or frozen florets. The gentle cooking process preserves the antioxidant power of these tasty cruciferous vegetables.

Makes: 4 servings
Active Time: 15 minutes
Total Time: 30 minutes

1 tablespoon rapeseed oil
1 small red onion, sliced in rings
½ teaspoon salt
¼ teaspoon freshly ground black pepper
700 g (1 lb 9 oz) romanesco florets
½ teaspoon curry powder (optional)
910 ml (32 fl oz) chicken stock
125 g (4½ oz) mascarpone

1. Heat a pan over high heat. Add the oil, onions, salt, and pepper. Immediately reduce the heat to medium and cook for 4–5 minutes, stirring occasionally, until the onions turn golden yellow. Add the romanesco and curry powder, if using. Cook for 1 minute more, stirring often, until the curry powder becomes fragrant.
2. Add the chicken stock plus 240 ml (8 fl oz) of water. Bring to the boil, then reduce the heat to a simmer, cover and cook 5–6 minutes, until the vegetables are tender. Turn off the heat and stir in the mascarpone. Purée with hand-held blender until smooth, or transfer to a blender to purée. Serve immediately.

PER SERVING: Net Carbs: 4 grams; Fibre: 2 grams; Protein: 7 grams; Fat: 30 grams; Calories: 313; Foundation Vegetables Net Carbs: 3 grams

VARIATIONS

- Use a combination of broccoli, Chinese cabbage, and/or asparagus instead of romanesco.
- Substitute cream cheese, soured cream, or double cream for the mascarpone.

No-Bean Chicken Chilli

This chilli is pale in colour, thanks to shredded chicken spiked with lime and cauliflower, but it has big, bold flavours – no beans about it! Cooking the chicken with its skin and bones yields superior flavour and keeps the meat from drying out. Letting it rest in the stock finishes the cooking without toughening the meat, as boiling does. This dish freezes well, so feel free to double the recipe.

Makes: 4 servings
Active Time: 10 minutes
Total Time: 45 minutes

3 chicken breasts, with bones and skin
½ teaspoon mild chilli powder
¼ teaspoon salt
1 tablespoon butter
½ small red onion, chopped
1 red pepper, deseeded and chopped
325 g (11½ oz) cauliflower florets
910 ml (32 fl oz) chicken stock
2 limes, zest and juice (or 60 ml (2 fl oz) bottled lime juice)
125 ml (4 fl oz) soured cream
20 g (¾ oz) coriander, chopped

1. Season the chicken with chilli powder and salt. Heat a large pan over medium-high heat and add the butter. Add the chicken, skin side down, and cook 3–4 minutes, until brown. Turn. Add the onion, red pepper, and cauliflower. Cook for 2–3 minutes more, stirring the vegetables around the chicken.
2. Add the chicken stock and bring to a simmer over medium heat. Cover and cook 10 minutes, then turn off the heat and let rest for 30 minutes.

3. Remove the chicken from the soup. Remove and discard the skin. Shred the chicken and return it to the pan along with the lime zest and juice. Stir well.
4. To serve, top each bowl with a dollop of soured cream and scatter with chopped coriander.

> PER SERVING: Net Carbs: 5 grams; Fibre: 1 gram; Protein: 24 grams; Fat: 16 grams; Calories: 263; Foundation Vegetables Net Carbs: 3 grams

VARIATIONS

- Add 1 tablespoon chopped pickled jalapeño pepper or grated Cheddar cheese per serving.
- Replace the coriander with chopped parsley.
- Add colour and extra heat by replacing the soured cream with no-sugar-added salsa.
- Phases 2–4: Add 85 g (3 oz) tinned chickpeas, drained and rinsed.

Taco Soup

Beef, tomato, and chilli powder, the very ingredients used to stuff a taco, are at the heart of this savoury main-dish soup, which lends itself to numerous garnishes. Avoid stirring beef mince; searing it gives the meat a bit of crust that helps it remain in chunks instead of turning into fine shreds that can dry out. You can double this recipe and freeze leftovers in single portions.

Makes: 4 servings
Active Time: 10 minutes
Total Time: 30 minutes

1 tablespoon rapeseed oil
450 g (1 lb) beef mince
2 teaspoons mild or hot chilli powder
½ teaspoon ground cumin
¼ teaspoon salt
½ small red onion, finely chopped
1 small jalapeño, seeds removed and chopped
1 tablespoon tinned chipotle in adobo, chopped
910 ml (32 fl oz) beef or chicken stock
115 g (4 oz) tinned chopped tomatoes
325 g (11½ oz) cauliflower
225 g (8 oz) thinly sliced kale, stems and tough ribs removed
85 g (3 oz) pitted black olives, sliced
¼ teaspoon freshly ground black pepper

1. Heat a large pan over medium-high heat. Add the oil and beef. Without stirring, sear for 2–3 minutes. Sprinkle chilli powder, cumin, and salt over the beef, and stir once or twice. Add the onions, jalapeño, if using, and the chipotle in adobo and cook for 2–3 minutes more, until the beef has browned.
2. Lower the heat to medium and add the stock, chopped tomatoes, and cauliflower; simmer for 9–10 minutes. Add the kale and olives and cook for a further 2–3 minutes, until kale is soft. Season with pepper. Serve immediately.

PER SERVING: Net Carbs: 6 grams; Fibre: 2 grams; Protein: 29 grams; Fat: 19 grams; Calories: 317; Foundation Vegetables Net Carbs: 5 grams

VARIATIONS

- Replace beef mince with turkey mince.
- Phases 1–4 garnishes: grated cheese, chopped spring onions, pickled jalapeños, or soured cream.
- Phases 2–4 garnishes: cooked black or other beans, torn low-carb tortillas.
- Phases 3–4 garnishes: crumbled wholegrain tortilla chips.

Creamy Basil-Spinach Soup with Bacon Bits ◔

This elegant, bright green soup is incredibly easy to make but will make you look like a four-star chef! Spinach is a nutritional power-house, and its mild flavours go well with smoky bacon. Serve with a salad for a complete meal.

Makes: 4 servings
Active Time: 15 minutes
Total Time: 10 minutes

8 rashers smoked bacon
1 tablespoon virgin olive oil
½ small red onion, chopped
910 ml (32 fl oz) chicken or beef stock
140 g (5 oz) baby spinach
60 g (2¼ oz) fresh basil leaves, plus 4 sprigs for garnish
¼ teaspoon freshly ground black pepper
125 g (4½ oz) mascarpone

1. Put the bacon rashers in a large cold frying pan. Place over medium heat and cook for 5–6 minutes, turning often, until crisp. Transfer to a plate covered with kitchen paper to drain. Set aside.
2. Warm the olive oil in a large pan over medium heat. Add onion and cook for 4–5 minutes, stirring often, until soft. Turn the heat down to low and add the stock. Add the spinach, basil, black pepper, and mascarpone. Purée using a hand-held blender, or transfer to a blender and process until smooth.
3. Divide the soup into four bowls and crumble two bacon rashers over each bowl. Top each with a sprig of basil and serve immediately, or refrigerate and serve chilled.

PER SERVING: Net Carbs: 4 grams; Fibre: 2 grams; Protein: 13 grams; Fat: 37 grams; Calories: 389; Foundation Vegetables Net Carbs: 3 grams

VARIATIONS

- Use watercress instead of baby spinach.
- Use defrosted frozen spinach instead of baby spinach and cook for an additional minute.

- Use cream cheese, soured cream, or double cream instead of mascarpone.
- After two weeks in Induction, top with a handful of toasted walnuts and use vegetable stock instead of beef or chicken.

Salmon Mushroom Chowder

This creamy chowder will remind you of holidays at the seaside! Mushrooms replace the usual high-carb potatoes. A small amount of coconut flour thickens the stock with a minimum of carbs. Don't forget the seafood seasoning, which flavours this otherwise mild chowder. Your fishmonger may be willing to cut up the salmon for chowder. Buying sliced mushrooms will save you a few more precious minutes.

Makes: 4 servings
Active Time: 10 minutes
Total Time: 20 minutes

1 tablespoon butter
2 celery sticks, chopped
225 g (8 oz) white or cremini mushrooms, sliced
½ small red onion, finely chopped
½ teaspoon Old Bay (available online or from some supermarkets and delis) or other seafood seasoning
¼ teaspoon freshly ground black pepper
3 tablespoons coconut flour
450 ml (16 fl oz) chicken stock
450 g (1 lb) fresh salmon, cut in 2.5-cm (1-in) chunks
125 ml (4 fl oz) double cream
100 g (3½ oz) Cheddar cheese, grated
1 tablespoon chopped parsley

1. In a large pan heat the butter over medium-low heat. Add the celery, mushrooms, onion, seafood seasoning, and black pepper; cook, stirring, for 5–6 minutes, until the celery is tender. Stir in the coconut flour until it coats the vegetables. Stir in chicken stock. Bring to a simmer over medium heat, stirring frequently.

2. Add the salmon and cook for 2–3 minutes, until the fish is cooked through but not overcooked. Add the cream and cheese and cook, stirring, until the cheese has melted and the soup just begins to bubble. Divide the soup into four bowls, garnish with parsley, and serve immediately.

PER SERVING: Net Carbs: 6 grams; Fibre: 3 grams; Protein: 34 grams; Fat: 39 grams; Calories: 524: Foundation Vegetables Net Carbs: 3 grams

VARIATIONS

- Replace salmon with tilapia or cod. Decrease the cooking time by 1 minute after adding the fish to the stock.
- Use tinned salmon (remove the skin and bones) or vacuum-packed salmon instead of fresh salmon. Add it after the cream and cheese, and just heat through.

SNACKS

Mozzarella Sticks

Gooey melted cheese inside a crunchy crust – what could be more irresistible? Here's another low-carb "interpretation" of a typically high-carb snack. Instead of breading, the sticks are coated in ground flaxseed.

Makes: 6 (2-stick) servings
Active Time: 10 minutes
Total Time: 1 hour

40 g (1½ oz) ground flaxseed
25 g (1 oz) grated Parmesan cheese
2 tablespoons finely chopped parsley
1 teaspoon garlic powder
½ teaspoon baking powder
450 g (1 lb) shredded mozzarella
325 g (11½ oz) cooked and roughly chopped cauliflower
1 large egg
Rapeseed oil or olive oil cooking spray
1 tablespoon rapeseed oil or high-oleic safflower oil
6 tablespoons no-sugar-added tomato sauce

1. Place the flaxseed, Parmesan, parsley, garlic powder, and baking powder on a sheet of greaseproof paper. Mix with your fingertips or a spoon.
2. Place the mozzarella and chopped cauliflower in a large bowl and mix well. Take 1 heaping tablespoon of the mixture and, using your fingers, form it into a 10-cm (4-in) long stick. Place on a plate. Repeat with remaining cauliflower-cheese mixture. You should get 12 sticks.
3. Whisk the egg in a shallow bowl.
4. Dip each stick in the whisked egg and then roll in the flaxseed-Parmesan mixture. Repeat, placing each on a freezer-safe plate. Cover with cling film and freeze for 30 minutes (or more) to firm before frying.

THE NEW ATKINS MADE EASY

5. When ready to serve, coat a large frying pan with cooking spray and heat over high heat. Add the oil. Add the sticks and cook for a total of 4–5 minutes, turning once or twice and coating with another layer of the cooking spray. Serve immediately with hot tomato sauce.

> PER SERVING: Net Carbs: 3 grams; Fibre: 2 grams; Protein: 12 grams; Fat: 14 grams; Calories: 195; Foundation Vegetables Net Carbs: 2 grams

VARIATIONS

- If the mozzarella sticks are completely frozen, preheat the oven to 200°C (400°F). Cook them according to the directions in Step 5, then slide the frying pan into the oven and bake for 5–6 minutes, until cooked through. Serve immediately.
- Replace the bottled tomato sauce with Fast, Spicy, Smooth Tomato Sauce (page 235).

Crunchy Asiago Crackers ◐ ▤

These crackers rely on two kinds of cheese and ground flaxseed instead of grains. Aged Asiago cheese resembles Parmesan but is moister and milder (you can find it in some cheese shops and Italian delis). These crackers also make a great topping for most soups. Make the cracker batter up to eight hours ahead and store in the refrigerator. Wrap leftover crackers in cling film and keep at room temperature for up to 3 days.

Makes: 4 servings (20 crackers)
Active Time: 10 minutes
Total Time: 20 minutes

55 g (2 oz) finely grated aged Asiago cheese
55 g (2 oz) shredded mozzarella
40 g (1½ oz) ground flaxseed
1 tablespoon finely chopped parsley
1 tablespoon sesame seeds (optional)
½ teaspoon garlic powder
½ teaspoon chilli powder
Rapeseed oil or olive oil cooking spray

1. Preheat oven to (200°C) 400°F and place the rack in the middle. Cover a large baking sheet with baking parchment.
2. Place the Asiago, mozzarella, flaxseed, parsley, sesame seeds, if using, garlic powder, and chilli powder in a large bowl. Mix well with a spoon. (If the mixture seems too dry, add ½ teaspoon water.) Place 1 tablespoon of the mixture in your palm. Press into a disk and place on the baking sheet. Continue, making 20 disks and spacing them 5 cm (2 inch) apart.
3. Coat the back of a spoon with cooking spray and press the crackers flat. Bake 8–9 minutes, until crisp and lightly browned. Transfer to a plate to cool. Serve immediately.

PER SERVING: Net Carbs: 1 gram; Fibre: 3 grams; Protein: 8 grams; Fat: 12 grams; Calories: 149; Foundation Vegetables Net Carbs: 0 grams

VARIATIONS

- Use Parmesan in place of Asiago cheese.
- Instead of sesame seeds, use 1 tablespoon finely chopped pumpkin seeds.

Crispy Kale Chips

A "superfood", kale turns up in salads, soups, and all sorts of other dishes. But who would have thought that kale could make a great low-carb stand-in for crisps, popcorn, or pretzels? You can go to health food shops and spend a bundle for a little bag of these savoury treats, or you make them yourself in a few minutes for a lot less money. Be sure to massage oil into the kale to make the chips crispy instead of greasy.

Makes: 4 servings
Active Time: 5 minutes
Total Time: 15 minutes

140 g (5 oz) curly kale, stems and tough ribs removed
2 teaspoons virgin olive oil
Pinch salt
2 tablespoons ground flaxseed
2 teaspoons sesame seeds
2 tablespoons grated Cheddar cheese

1. Preheat the oven to 200°C (400°F). Wash the kale, tear into 10-cm (4-in) wide pieces, and dry well with kitchen paper so that it will crisp better when baked.
2. Transfer the strips of kale to a large bowl and scatter over the olive oil. Using your fingertips, rub the olive oil into the kale leaves until coated. Sprinkle with the salt, flaxseed, and sesame seeds. Spread the kale out on an ungreased baking sheet. Sprinkle evenly with the cheese and bake 10–12 minutes, until the kale is crisp and the cheese has melted.
3. Serve immediately, or store in an airtight container at room temperature for up to three days.

PER SERVING: Net Carbs: 3 grams; Fibre: 2 grams; Protein: 3 grams; Fat: 5 grams; Calories: 68; Foundation Vegetables Net Carbs: 3 grams

Courgette Parmesan Fritters

These cheesy, herb-filled fritters would also work well topped with smoked salmon as part of a brunch menu.

Makes: 6 servings (12 fritters)
Active Time: 10 minutes
Total Time: 20 minutes

4 large eggs, separated
2 medium courgettes, trimmed and grated
55 g (2 oz) grated Parmesan cheese
55 g (2 oz) shredded mozzarella
15 g (½ oz) fresh parsley, chopped
15 g (½ oz) fresh basil, chopped
40 g (1½ oz) coconut-flax flour blend
½ teaspoon baking powder
⅛ teaspoon ground nutmeg
¼ teaspoon salt
Rapeseed oil or olive oil cooking spray
3 teaspoons rapeseed oil or virgin olive oil

1. Place the egg whites in a large bowl and whisk using an electric mixer, until stiff peaks form. Set aside.
2. Place the egg yolks, grated courgette, Parmesan, mozzarella, parsley, basil, coconut-flax flour blend, baking powder, nutmeg, and salt in another large bowl. Stir well until the courgette is well coated with the mixture. Using a spatula, gently fold in the egg whites until just combined. There will be streaks of egg white.
3. Coat a large frying pan with cooking spray. Warm the frying pan over medium-high heat and add 1 teaspoon oil. Using a large serving spoon as a measure, pour out four fritters. Cook 2–3 minutes on each side, until lightly browned. Transfer to a plate. Repeat twice, using 1 teaspoon of oil and four measures of batter each time.
4. Serve immediately or refrigerate, covered with cling film, and reheat when ready to serve.

PER SERVING: Net Carbs: 3 grams; Fibre: 2 grams; Protein: 11 grams; Fat: 11 grams; Calories: 159; Foundation Vegetables Net Carbs: 2 grams

VARIATION

• Use 40 g (1½ oz) ground flaxseed instead of the coconut-flax flour blend.

Prawn Cocktail with Lemony Garlic Sauce ◑ ▤

If you use cooked fresh or frozen prawns, this new take on prawn cocktail just requires assembly. If you purchase frozen prawns, select medium or large ones. The small ones tend to get waterlogged and don't defrost as well. Make the dipping sauce early in the day and refrigerate.

Makes: 6 servings
Active Time: 5 minutes
Total Time: 10 minutes

1 lemon, zest and juice
   (or 2 tablespoons bottled lemon juice)
30 g (1 oz) feta cheese
3 garlic cloves, finely chopped
½ teaspoon Dijon mustard
½ teaspoon Worcestershire sauce
2 tablespoons extra-virgin olive oil
1 teaspoon Tabasco or other hot sauce
¼ teaspoon salt
¼ teaspoon black pepper
450 g (1 lb) peeled and cooked fresh or
   defrosted prawns

1. Place the lemon zest and juice, feta, garlic, mustard, Worcestershire sauce, olive oil, hot sauce, salt, pepper, and 50 ml (2 fl oz) of water in a blender or food processor. Process until smooth.
2. Top each prawn cocktail serving with 2 tablespoons of sauce.

PER SERVING: Net Carbs: 3 grams; Fibre: 0 grams; Protein: 18 grams; Fat: 7 grams; Calories: 151; Foundation Vegetables Net Carbs: 0 grams

VARIATIONS

- Serve the sauce over leftover flank steak from the recipe for Crisp Lettuce Wedge with Sliced Flank Steak (page 241) or as a dip with raw broccoli.
- Use the sauce as a dip for grilled or barbecued skewered chicken, raw courgette sticks, sliced red peppers, and radishes. They make a great picnic treat.

DESSERTS

Fudgy Ice Lollies

You may need to hide these from your kids! Better yet, make a double batch, but don't reveal the secret ingredient: spinach. The flavour is masked by cocoa. No ice lolly moulds handy? Use disposable small paper or plastic cups or even small clean yoghurt pots, and insert a lightweight plastic spoon.

Makes: 4 servings
Active Time: 10 minutes
Total Time: 4 hours and
　　　　　 10 minutes

125 ml (4 fl oz) double cream
2 tablespoons unsweetened cocoa powder
½ teaspoon cinnamon (optional)
1 teaspoon vanilla extract
4 teaspoons acceptable sweetener
30 g (1 oz) packed fresh baby spinach leaves

1. Place cream, cocoa powder, cinnamon, if using, vanilla, sweetener, spinach, and 175 ml (6 fl oz) of water in a blender and process until very smooth.
2. Pour into ice lolly moulds and freeze at least 4 hours before serving. To remove from the moulds, run the moulds under hot water for 30 seconds, or simply leave the lollies on the work surface for 30 minutes before serving to soften them enough for easy release.

PER SERVING: Net Carbs: 3 grams; Fibre: 1 gram; Protein: 1 gram; Fat: 12 grams; Calories: 118; Foundation Vegetables Net Carbs: 0 grams

VARIATIONS

- Instead of cinnamon, add ¼ teaspoon almond extract or a pinch of cayenne.
- Phases 2–4: Add 60 ml (2 fl oz) bourbon or whisky for adult ice lollies.

Devil's Food Panna Cotta

Italian for "cooked cream", panna cotta is a dessert made in heaven for Atkins followers. Be sure the water in which you place the gelatine is cold or the gelatine won't "bloom". You can also use sheet gelatine; just follow the instructions on the packet.

Makes: 4 servings
Active Time: 10 minutes
Total Time: 2 hours 10 minutes

4 teaspoons unflavoured gelatine
175 ml (6 fl oz) single cream
2 tablespoons unsweetened cocoa powder
1 teaspoon acceptable sweetener
1 teaspoon instant coffee
1 teaspoon vanilla extract

1. Place four 100-ml (3½-fl oz) ramekins on a large plate. Refrigerate while you prepare the panna cotta.
2. Place 175 ml (6 fl oz) cold water in a small pan. Sprinkle with gelatine; let stand until gelatine has softened, about 5 minutes. Do not stir. Place over low heat and cook for 1 minute, stirring well until the gelatine dissolves. Pour into a blender.
3. Add the cream, cocoa powder, sweetener, coffee, and vanilla extract. Blend until smooth.
4. Pour mixture into the 4 chilled ramekins. Cover with cling film and refrigerate on the plate until set, about 2 hours. Store up to 3 days, covered, in the refrigerator.

PER SERVING: Net Carbs: 3 grams; Fibre: 1 gram; Protein: 4 grams; Fat: 6 grams; Calories: 77; Foundation Vegetables Net Carbs: 0 grams

VARIATIONS

- Top with 1 tablespoon unsweetened whipping cream or drizzle with sugar-free chocolate or vanilla syrup.
- After two weeks in Phase 1: Top with 1 tablespoon toasted and chopped hazelnuts or walnuts.

Tiramisu ◑ ▤

Our low-carb spin on this classic Italian pudding eliminates the sponge fingers but keeps the complex flavour. Be sure the soya milk–gelatine mixture is cool, otherwise the fat in the mascarpone will solidify and the pudding will separate.

Makes: 4 servings
Active Time: 15 minutes
Total Time: 2 hours, 15 minutes

2 teaspoons instant coffee
1 tablespoon acceptable sweetener
8 teaspoons sugar-free chocolate syrup
225 ml (8 fl oz) plain unsweetened soya milk
1 teaspoon unflavoured gelatine
250 g (9 oz) mascarpone
1 teaspoon vanilla extract
½ teaspoon unsweetened cocoa powder

1. Place 2 teaspoons water in a small bowl with instant coffee and sweetener. Whisk well to combine. Stir in the chocolate syrup. Divide the mixture among four ramekins or parfait glasses.
2. Place 60 ml (2 fl oz) of the soya milk in a small saucepan. Sprinkle with gelatine; let stand until the gelatine has softened, about 5 minutes. Do not stir. Place over low heat and cook 1 minute, stirring well, until the gelatine dissolves.
3. Turn off the heat. Cool the soya-gelatin mixture 5 minutes or until it reaches room temperature. Whisk in the remaining soya milk, mascarpone, and vanilla until smooth.
4. Divide the mascarpone mixture among the four ramekins; the syrup mixture creates a swirl as you pour. Refrigerate, uncovered, for at least 2 hours. Sprinkle ⅛ teaspoon cocoa over each pudding and serve, or store covered for up to 3 days in the fridge.

PER SERVING: Net Carbs: 3 grams; Fibre: 1 gram; Protein: 7 grams; Fat: 25 grams; Calories: 273; Foundation Vegetables Net Carbs: 0 grams

VARIATIONS

- Instead of refrigerating in ramekins, freeze the pudding mixture in ice lolly moulds.
- Instead of soya milk, use plain no-sugar-added almond milk or coconut milk beverage.
- Instead of sugar-free chocolate syrup, use hazelnut, caramel, or raspberry syrup.
- Top with shaved sugar-free dark chocolate.
- Phases 2–4: Stir in a few raspberries.

Lemon Crêpes

Crêpes use more liquid and eggs than pancakes do, making them thinner and less dense. Since the batter doesn't freeze well, make all the crêpes and keep leftovers for up to four days in the refrigerator.

Makes: 6 servings (12 crêpes)
Active Time: 15 minutes
Total Time: 25 minutes

4 large eggs, separated
¼ teaspoon salt
175 ml (6 fl oz) plain unsweetened soya milk
125 g (4½ oz) mascarpone
2 tablespoons butter, melted and cooled
1 lemon, zest and juice
1 tablespoon acceptable sweetener
1 teaspoon vanilla extract
40 g (1½ oz) coconut-flax flour blend
2 tablespoons plain unsweetened protein powder
1 teaspoon baking powder
Rapeseed oil or olive oil cooking spray
3 teaspoons rapeseed oil

1. Place the egg whites and salt in a large mixing bowl and whisk using an electric mixer until stiff peaks form. Set aside.
2. Place the egg yolks, soya milk, mascarpone, butter, lemon juice and zest, sweetener, and vanilla in another large bowl. Whisk until

well combined. Add the coconut-flax flour blend, protein powder, and baking powder. Add a large spoonful of beaten egg white. Using a spatula, fold the dry ingredients and egg white into the mixture until just combined and a sticky mass forms. Add another large spoonful of egg white and fold again until the mixture becomes lighter. Fold in the remaining egg white. Don't overmix; there will be small lumps.

3. Coat a large frying pan with cooking spray. Place over high heat and add 1 teaspoon rapeseed oil. Using a large serving spoon as a measure, drop four spoonfuls of batter onto the heated pan and spread out with the back of a spoon. Cook until the bottom is firm, about 3–5 minutes. Flip and press lightly with the spatula. Cook another 1–2 minutes, until crêpes are cooked through. Transfer to a plate. Repeat twice with remaining rapeseed oil and crêpe batter. Serve immediately.

PER SERVING: Net Carbs: 2 grams; Fibre: 2 grams; Protein: 11 grams; Fat: 20 grams; Calories: 243; Foundation Vegetables Net Carbs: 0 grams

VARIATIONS

- Substitute 40 g (1½ oz) finely ground flaxseed for the coconut-flax flour blend.
- Fill each crêpe with 1 tablespoon unsweetened whipping cream, with or without a splash of sugar-free flavoured syrup or some grated sugar-free chocolate.
- Phases 2–4: Fill with fresh berries or 1 tablespoon no-sugar-added preserves. Or fill with whipping cream flavoured with a splash of bourbon or whisky.

Green Tea Slushie

If you enjoy green tea ice cream, this slushie will become your new favourite. Green tea powder (also called matcha) can be found in supermarkets. You can also find it at Asian markets and health food shops, or order it online. Double the recipe if you wish.

Makes: 2 servings
Active Time: 5 minutes
Total Time: 10 minutes

225 ml (8 fl oz) plain unsweetened soya milk
60 ml (2 fl oz) double cream
about 8 ice cubes
1 teaspoon acceptable sweetener
1 teaspoon vanilla extract
1 teaspoon green tea powder

1. Place all the ingredients in a blender and process until smooth.
2. Pour into two parfait or other tall glasses and serve immediately.

PER SERVING: Net Carbs: 3 grams; Fibre: 1 gram; Protein: 4 grams; Fat: 13 grams; Calories: 152; Foundation Vegetables Net Carbs: 0 grams

VARIATIONS

- Replace soya milk with plain unsweetened almond milk or coconut milk beverage.
- Add ¼ teaspoon mint extract and 1 tablespoon sugar-free chocolate chips.
- Replace the green tea powder with 1 teaspoon instant coffee.
- Serve with a drizzle of sugar-free chocolate syrup.

AFTERWORD

Jeff S. Volek, PhD, RD

THE SCIENCE SUPPORTING ATKINS

I can virtually guarantee that you will be astonished when you hear about the current science supporting Atkins, especially the evolving new lines of research. The New Atkins Diet won't merely help you lose weight; in fact, that's just the tip of the iceberg. This chapter will provide a snapshot of the existing science supporting Atkins, as well as an overview of the emerging research on exciting new applications of a low-carbohydrate lifestyle. I have no doubt that after reading this chapter, you'll be confident that this is the best approach for lifelong health and wellness.

WHY ATKINS WORKS BETTER THAN OTHER APPROACHES

The number one reason why the New Atkins Diet works so well is that it targets the fundamental problem most overweight people experience. That problem is insulin resistance. Simply put, if you have insulin resistance, and many millions of people do, you don't metabolise dietary carbohydrate in an efficient way. Rather than burn carbohydrate for fuel, you tend to tuck it away as body fat. In fact, you are intolerant to sugars and starches. If you are carbohydrate-intolerant, then it makes sense to limit sugars and starches; this is the cornerstone of the New Atkins Diet. When people who are carb-intolerant follow Atkins, they experience amazing improvements in their health. Their metabolism shifts to burning mainly fat, which causes increased circulating levels of specific metabolites called ketones. Ketones are the preferred fuel for the brain and other tissues, and are being studied for a range of therapeutic applications. Running on a fat-burning metabolism is associated with higher energy levels, reduced carb cravings, higher satiety, and nearly effortless weight loss.

The science supporting Atkins goes back to at least the middle of the last century, but it has really picked up during the last decade. We now have a much better understanding of how and why controlling carbohydrates works to melt away fat and fend off diabetes, heart disease, cancer, and a host of other diseases.

WEIGHT-LOSS STUDIES

There have been a large number of studies comparing weight-loss responses between low-carbohydrate and low-fat diets, ranging from a few weeks to as long as two years. It's clear that, on average, following the Atkins Diet results in greater weight loss than other approaches higher in carbohydrate content. When you specifically look at those studies where the low-carb diet resembled Atkins and there was good compliance to the diet protocols, the results are nothing short of dramatic. For example, when my associates and I had 40 overweight men and women consume either an Atkins-like diet or a low-fat diet for 12 weeks, the average weight loss was twice as much on Atkins (10 kg /22 lb versus 5 kg/11 lb).[1] Weight loss varied significantly among participants, but the average loss for those on Atkins was greater than the loss by any single person on the low-fat diet. **And when we X-rayed participants to determine body composition, we saw that those following Atkins had lost more total fat and specifically more belly fat.** Why does the Atkins Diet work so well for promoting weight and fat loss? This is still an open question among researchers, but the most likely reason is that restricting carbohydrates increases satiety, making it easier to restrict calories.

METABOLIC SYNDROME

Approximately one in ten adults in the United States has diabetes, and one in three has metabolic syndrome (pre-diabetes). A primary application of very low-carbohydrate diets in adults is to manage insulin-resistant conditions. Insulin resistance (carbohydrate intolerance) is the hallmark of Type 2 diabetes and is also the primary defect underlying metabolic syndrome. Like other food intolerances, the most logical and effective approach to managing carbohydrate intolerance is to restrict the offending nutrient. To get right to the point, the Atkins Diet is a highly potent therapy for managing pre-diabetes and Type 2 diabetes. In fact, it's many times more potent and safer, than any medications for treating these conditions. Not only can the Atkins Diet prevent Type 2 diabetes and slow down its progression, but it can also actually resolve all the signs and symptoms of the disease, in effect putting it into remission permanently.

What is the evidence for such powerful statements? First let's take an overview of the work on metabolic syndrome, and then we'll look at the key studies performed on individuals with Type 2 diabetes. Metabolic syndrome is best described as pre-diabetes and provides an early sign the body is struggling to manage dietary carbohydrate in a healthy way. The main features of metabolic syndrome are excessive belly fat; high blood levels of glucose, insulin, and triglycerides; low HDL cholesterol; and high blood pressure. You don't have to have all these signs, but if you have more than two, then you have metabolic syndrome. Studies estimate that approximately 64 million Americans have metabolic syndrome.[2] You have metabolic syndrome if at least three of the following are present:

- Waist circumference: ≥ 101 cm (40 in) (men) or ≥ 89 cm (35 in) (women)
- Fasting triglycerides: ≥150 mg/dL
- HDL cholesterol: < 40 mg/dL (men) or < 50 mg/dL (women)
- Blood pressure: ≥ 130/85 mm Hg or use of high blood pressure medication
- Fasting glucose: ≥ 100 mg/dL or use of hyperglycaemia medication.

The primary driver of metabolic syndrome is consumption of more sugars and starches than an individual can tolerate. A large number of studies have shown that the features of metabolic syndrome dramatically improve with carbohydrate restriction.[3] In fact, the Atkins Diet improves all the signs and symptoms of metabolic syndrome, often in dramatic fashion. Take, for example, the study in which my colleagues and I compared the Atkins Diet to a standard American diet in individuals with metabolic syndrome.[4] After three months, individuals in both groups lost weight, but weight loss and fat loss, including belly fat, were greater with the Atkins Diet. In the participants on the Atkins Diet, blood triglycerides plummeted by 51 per cent, HDL ("good") cholesterol increased by 11 per cent, and insulin sensitivity improved by 55 per cent; there were even significant reductions in low-grade inflammation and functioning of blood vessels. This and many other studies clearly show the Atkins Diet is superior to low-fat/high carbohydrate diets for managing metabolic syndrome.

TYPE 2 DIABETES

What if you have progressed past metabolic syndrome and have Type 2 diabetes? The Atkins Diet could actually reverse your situation. Going back almost four decades, researchers have noted that Type 2 diabetics consuming a very low-calorie carbohydrate-restricted diet experienced major weight loss (even as they retained muscle mass), saw improvements in blood cholesterol and blood pressure, and could discontinue their diabetic medication.[5] Two decades later, an even more provocative study was published, showing that improvement in diabetes is more dependent on carb restriction than calorie restriction and weight loss.[6] Obese Type 2 diabetics were fed two different diets, although both contained 650 calories a day, for three weeks. The two diets contained the same amount of protein but one consisted of 24 grams of carbohydrate per day, and the other 94 grams. The lower-carbohydrate diet resulted in significantly greater improvements in blood sugar control and sugar output by the liver. Interestingly, the magnitude of improvements was directly related to circulating ketone levels, indicating that the unique fat-burning state induced by the Atkins Diet specifically targets better diabetes management.

Ten years after that, it was shown that obese Type 2 diabetics following the Induction Phase of the Atkins Diet (20 grams of carbohydrate per day) had remarkable improvements in plasma glucose and haemoglobin A1c, and a 75 per cent increase in insulin sensitivity.[7]

These extraordinary effects were observed after only two weeks on the diet. There are also studies of longer duration. After more than one year of consuming an Atkins-like diet, Type 2 diabetics lost significant weight and had remarkable improvement in blood sugar (down 51 per cent), total cholesterol (down 29 per cent), HDL cholesterol (up 63 per cent), LDL cholesterol (down 33 per cent), and triglycerides (down 41 per cent).[8] Other studies also support the long-term efficacy of the Atkins Diet in managing complications of type 2 diabetes.[9-12]

IMPROVED BLOOD LIPIDS

Blood lipids are the substances that transport fats (triglycerides and cholesterol) through your bloodstream. Elevated levels of these fats in your blood can indicate a higher risk for heart disease. The ones most commonly measured are triglycerides and total cholesterol, which includes two types: LDL cholesterol and HDL cholesterol. Extensive research has shown that the Atkins Diet dependably improves all these lipid markers, and therefore reduces your risk of heart disease.[13] The most consistent response to restricting dietary carbohydrates is a decrease in circulating triglycerides. The effect can be quite potent, often slashing levels of triglycerides in half. After you eat a meal containing fat, blood triglycerides gradually increase and often stay elevated for several hours. The higher blood triglycerides go and the longer they stay elevated, the higher the risk for heart disease. After you have been on the Atkins Diet for several weeks, there is a dramatic improvement in your body's ability to process high-fat meals so fats don't accumulate in the blood.

As triglycerides plummet on the Atkins Diet, HDL usually increases. This is a positive response because HDL helps remove excess cholesterol from the body. The Atkins Diet does a better job at decreasing triglycerides while simultaneously increasing HDL than any other lifestyle factor, including exercise, and even outperforms most drugs.

In many cases, LDL will decrease or stay the same, but in some people it may increase. However, this variable response in LDL concentration from person to person is just part of the story. LDL particles come in different sizes, ranging from small to large. The Atkins

Diet consistently decreases the smaller LDL particles. These are the more dangerous ones, as they are significantly associated with heart disease.[14]

FATTY LIVER

The excess accumulation of fat in liver cells is tightly linked to over-consumption of carbohydrates, obesity, and insulin resistance (carbohydrate intolerance). Fatty liver significantly increases your risk of developing severe liver disease, diabetes, and heart disease. Fatty liver is not as simple to measure as BMI (body mass index) or blood cholesterol, and therefore statistics are not as precise, but it is estimated that between 20 million and 80 million Americans have this condition. Similar to its effect on improving diabetes, studies indicate that the Atkins Diet has a profound benefit on fatty liver.[15, 16] In one provocative study, obese men and women with fatty liver were fed either a low-fat or a low-carbohydrate Atkins-like diet. The low-fat diet contained slightly fewer calories and significantly more carbohydrate (169 grams a day) compared with the Atkins Diet (26 grams a day). Fatty liver was measured using sophisticated imaging techniques. Despite being higher in calories, after just two weeks the Atkins Diet led to significantly greater reductions in liver fat content.[16] This demonstrates that the Atkins Diet is a more effective treatment for fatty liver independent of weight loss.

WHAT ABOUT SATURATED FATS?

At this point you might be concerned about whether eating saturated fat on the Atkins Diet will affect your health. Fortunately, that has been the focus of rigorous research, and the results may shock you. Remember, the basic concept of the Atkins Diet is to reduce dietary carbohydrates to the point that you are able to preferentially burn your stored body fat as well as the fat you eat. It turns out that when you are on the Atkins Diet your body prefers to burn saturated fat for fuel. That means that the saturated fat you eat does not accumulate in your arteries or on your hips. Instead, it is promptly burned as fuel. Two studies have shown that levels of saturated fat in the blood actually go down in individuals consuming the Atkins Diet, whether or not they lost weight.[17, 18] This is an important effect of the Atkins Diet because people with higher levels of saturated fat in their blood have an increased risk of developing metabolic syndrome,[19] diabetes,[20] heart attack,[21] and heart failure.[22] The bottom line is that there is no need to fear or avoid saturated fat on the Atkins Diet; in fact, it provides a preferred fuel, adds flavour to food, and promotes satiety.

You might also be interested to learn that researchers are seriously reevaluating the saturated fat paradigm. **Large comprehensive reviews performed in recent years have all failed to find any association between saturated fat** intake and incidence of heart disease.[23, 24]

EPILEPSY AND OTHER NEUROLOGICAL DISEASES

Very low-carbohydrate diets have long been known to be an effective treatment for seizures. In many cases, such a diet can cure the disease within weeks, even in patients who fail to respond to epilepsy drugs.[25, 26] It is one of the more remarkable clinical benefits associated with the Atkins Diet. For children who are prone to seizures and who do not respond to medications, the diet is nothing short of a miracle. Although the medical literature is full of studies trying to understand how a low-carbohydrate, high-fat diet improves seizure control, it remains uncertain how exactly it works. The potent and rapidly expanding use of the Atkins Diet for treatment of epilepsy has inspired physicians and researchers to also study the effects of the diet on autism, brain tumours, and plaque development associated with Alzheimer's disease. Clinical trials are also under way on the use of low carbohydrate diets like Atkins on head trauma, stroke, Lou Gehrig's disease (ALS), and depression.

CANCER

Cancer is a mysterious and immensely complex disease, but emerging evidence links many types of cancer to the disturbed metabolic state observed in obesity. More specifically, the growth and progression of many cancers appear to be connected to higher intakes of carbohydrate and stimulation of insulin production. Since the Atkins Diet restricts carbohydrates and lowers insulin levels, often dramatically, it makes intuitive sense that it might be an effective treatment and preventative strategy for some, if not most, cancers. The metabolic state induced by the Atkins Diet, with low insulin and increased levels of ketones (the by-product of fat burning), has been linked to reduced tumour growth in animal studies of brain, prostate, colon, and breast cancer. Although the basic science looks promising, there have been few published human studies to date investigating the Atkins Diet on cancer progression. One recent pilot study in women with advanced breast cancer showed that the Atkins Diet stabilised and even decreased tumour glucose uptake.[27] There are, however, a growing number of case reports and pilot studies as well as several ongoing clinical trials, and the preliminary results that have been published or presented at conferences have been positive. Expect more comprehensive results soon as this relatively new application of the Atkins Diet gains traction.

THE NEXT FRONTIER

The science supporting Atkins for healthy weight loss is impressive, but equally exciting is the application in a number of other conditions. The Atkins Diet causes accelerated fat metabolism, which results in production of specific metabolites called ketones that are being studied in much greater detail as therapeutic agents. It turns out that when a person's (or an animal's) metabolism runs on these small molecules, there is a host of positive effects, including decreased oxidative stress and inflammatory markers and improved tolerance to stress. Besides the neurological diseases and cancers mentioned above, basic and applied scientists are studying the mechanisms of how this fat-burning state induced by the Atkins Diet improves wound healing, ameliorates post-traumatic stress disorder, slows down the aging process, and much more. Research is not just focused on weight loss and clinical applications. Recreational and elite athletes and soldiers are also using the Atkins Diet to enhance their physical and mental performance and speed recovery from exercise.

SUMMARY

There is already an impressive amount of research supporting the Atkins Diet for weight loss and metabolic health. The next decade will be enlightening as research continues to shed light on new applications. Because of the existing science and a long history of use, we can say with confidence that not only is the Atkins Diet safe, it's also a disease-fighting, health-promoting lifestyle.

• • •

Dr Volek is a professor in the number-one-ranked Department of Kinesiology at the University of Connecticut, where he teaches and leads a research team that explores the physiologic impact of various dietary and exercise regimes and nutritional supplements. Dr Volek's most significant line of work has been a series of studies performed over the last 15 years aimed at better understanding what constitutes a well-formulated low-carbohydrate diet and its impact on obesity, body composition, adaptations to training, and overall metabolic health. This line of work has shown profound effects of carbohydrate restriction on overall health and wellbeing, as well as on peak performance. He has published more than 250 scientific manuscripts and presented more than 100 talks at scientific and industry conferences in eight countries. Dr Volek is co-author of the *New York Times* bestselling *The New Atkins for a New You*, published in March 2010, and has subsequently self-published *The Art and Science of Low Carbohydrate Living* and *The Art and Science of Low Carbohydrate Performance*, which delve deeper into the science and application of low-carbohydrate diets.

NOTES

1. J. S. Volek, S. D. Phinney, C. E. Forsythe, E. E. Quann, R. J. Wood, M. J. Puglisi, et al, "Carbohydrate Restriction Has a More Favorable Impact on the Metabolic Syndrome Than a Low Fat Diet", *Lipids* 44(4) (2009), 297–309.
2. A. Mozumdar and G. Liguori, "Persistent Increase of Prevalence of Metabolic Syndrome Among U.S. Adults: NHANES III to NHANES 1999–2006", *Diabetes Care* 34(1) (2011), 216–219.
3. J. S. Volek and R. D. Feinman, "Carbohydrate Restriction Improves the Features of Metabolic Syndrome. Metabolic Syndrome may be defined by the response to carbohydrate restriction", *Nutrition & Metabolism* (London) 2 (2005), 31.
4. J. S. Volek, S. D. Phinney, C. E. Forsythe, E. E. Quann, R. J. Wood, M. J. Puglisi, et al, "Carbohydrate Restriction Has a More Favorable Impact on the Metabolic Syndrome Than a Low Fat Diet", *Lipids* 44(4) (2009), 297–309.
5. B. R. Bistrian, G. L. Blackburn, J. P. Flatt, J. Sizer, N. S. Scrimshaw, and M. Sherman, "Nitrogen Metabolism and Insulin Requirements in Obese Diabetic Adults on a Protein-sparing Modified Fast", *Diabetes* 25(6) (1976), 494–504.
6. B. Gumbiner, J. A. Wendel, and M. P. McDermott, "Effects of Diet Composition and Ketosis on Glycemia During Very-Low-Energy-Diet Therapy in Obese Patients with Non-Insulin-Dependent Diabetes Mellitus", *American Journal of Clinical Nutrition* 63(1) (1996), 110–15.

7. G. Boden, K. Sargrad, C. Homko, M. Mozzoli, and T. P. Stein, "Effect of a Low-Carbohydrate Diet on Appetite, Blood Glucose Levels, and Insulin Resistance in Obese Patients with type 2 Diabetes", *Annals of Internal Medicine* 142 (2005), 403–411.

8. H. M. Dashti, N. S. Al-Zaid, T. C. Mathew, M. Al-Mousawi, H. Talib, S. K. Asfar, and A. I. Behbahani, "Long Term Effects of Ketogenic Diet in Obese Subjects with High Cholesterol Level", *Molecular and Cellular Biochemistry* 286 (2006), 1–9.

9. W. S. Yancy Jr., M. Foy, A. M. Chalecki, M. C. Vernon, and E. C. Westman, "A Low-Carbohydrate, Ketogenic Diet to Treat type 2 Diabetes", Nutrition & Metabolism (London) 2 (2005), 34.

10. J. V. Nielsen and E. A. Joensson, "Low-Carbohydrate Diet in type 2 Diabetes: Stable Improvement of Bodyweight and Glycemic Control During 44 Months Follow-Up", *Nutrition & Metabolism* (London) 5 (2008), 14.

11. T. A. Hussain, T. C. Mathew, A. A. Dashti, S. Asfar, N. Al-Zaid, and H. M. Dashti, "Effect of Low-Calorie Versus Low-Carbohydrate Ketogenic Diet in type 2 Diabetes", *Nutrition* 10 (2012), 1016–1021.

12. J. S. Volek, M. J. Sharman, and C. E. Forsythe, "Modification of Lipoproteins by Very Low-Carbohydrate Diets", *The Journal of Nutrition* 135 (2005), 1339–1342.

13. B. Lamarche, I. Lemieux, and J. P. Despres, "The Small, Dense LDL Phenotype and the Risk of Coronary Heart Disease: Epidemiology, Patho-Physiology and Therapeutic Aspects", *Diabetes & Metabolism* 1999; 25(3), 199–211.

14. K. El Harchaoui, et al., "Value of Low-Density Lipoprotein Particle Number and Size as Predictors of Coronary Artery Disease in Apparently Healthy Men and Women: the EPIC-Norfolk Prospective Population Study", *Journal of the American College of Cardiology* 49(5) (2007), 547–553.

15. D. Tendler, S. Lin, W. S. Yancy Jr., J. Mavropoulos, P. Sylvestre, D. C. Rockey, and E. C. Westman, "The Effect of a Low-Carbohydrate, Ketogenic Diet on Nonalcoholic Fatty Liver Disease: A Pilot Study", *Digestive Diseases and Sciences* 52(2) (2007): 589–93.

16. J. D. Browning, J. A. Baker, T. Rogers, J. Davis, S. Satapati, and S. C. Burgess, "Short-Term Weight Loss and Hepatic Triglyceride

Reduction: Evidence of a Metabolic Advantage with Dietary Carbohydrate Restriction", *American Journal of Clinical Nutrition* 93(5) (2011), 1048–1052.

17. C. E. Forsythe, S. D. Phinney, M. L. Fernandez, E. E. Quann, R. J. Wood, D. M. Bibus, et. al., "Comparison of Low Fat and Low Carbohydrate Diets on Circulating Fatty Acid Composition and Markers of Inflammation", *Lipids* 43(1) (2008), 65–77.

18. C.E.Forsythe,S.D.Phinney,R.D.Feinman,B.M.Volk,D.Freidenreich, E. Quann, K. Ballard, M. J. Puglisi, C. M. Maresh, W. J. Kraemer, et al., "Limited Effect of Dietary Saturated Fat on Plasma Saturated Fat in the Context of a Low Carbohydrate Diet", *Lipids* 45(10) (2010), 947–962.

19. E. Warensjo, R. Riserus, and B. Vessby, "Fatty Acid Composition of Serum Lipids Predicts the Development of the Metabolic Syndrome in Men", *Diabetologia* 48(10) (2005), 1999–2005.

20. P. S. Patel, S. J. Sharp, E. Jansen, R. N. Luben, K. T. Khaw, N. J. Wareham, and N. G. Forouhi, "Fatty Acids Measured in Plasma and Erythrocyte-Membrane Phospholipids and Derived by Food-Frequency Questionnaire and the Risk of New-Onset type 2 Diabetes: A Pilot Study in the European Prospective Investigation into Cancer and Nutrition (EPIC)-Norfolk cohort", *American Journal of Clinical Nutrition* 92(5) (2010), 1214–1222.

21. L. Wang, A. R. Folsom, and J. H. Eckfeldt, "Plasma Fatty Acid Composition and Incidence of Coronary Heart Disease in Middle Aged Adults: The Atherosclerosis Risk in Communities (ARIC) Study", *Nutrition, Metabolism & Cardiovascular Diseases* 13(5) (2003), 256–266.

22. K. Yamagishi, H. Iso, H. Yatsuya, N. Tanabe, C. Date, S. Kikuchi, A. Yamamoto, Y. Inaba, and A. Tamakoshi, "Dietary Intake of Saturated Fatty Acids and Mortality from Cardiovascular Disease in Japanese: The Japan Collaborative Cohort Study for Evaluation of Cancer Risk (JACC) Study", *American Journal of Clinical Nutrition* 92(4) (2010), 759–765.

23. M. U. Jakobsen, E. J. O'Reilly, B. L. Heitmann, M. A. Pereira, K. Balter, G. E. Fraser, U. Goldbourt, G. Hallmans, P. Knekt, S. Liu, et al, "Major Types of Dietary Fat and Risk of Coronary Heart Disease: A Pooled Analysis of 11 Cohort Studies", *American Journal of Clinical Nutrition* 89(5) (2009), 1425–1432.

24.P. W. Siri-Tarino, Q. Sun, F. B. Hu, and R. M. Krauss, "Meta-Analysis of Prospective Cohort Studies Evaluating the Association of Saturated Fat with Cardiovascular Disease", *American Journal of Clinical Nutrition* 91(3) (2010), 535–546.

25.E. H. Kossoff, and J. L. Dorward, "The Modified Atkins Diet", *Epilepsia* 49 Suppl 8 (2008), 37–41.

26.E. H. Kossoff et al, "Optimal Clinical Management of Children Receiving the Ketogenic Diet: Recommendations of the International Ketogenic Diet Study Group", *Epilepsia* 50(2) (2009), 304–317.

27.E. J. Fine, C. J. Segal-Isaacson, R. D. Feinman, S. Herszkopf, M. C. Romano, N. Tomuta, A. F. Bontempo, N. Negassa, and J. A. Sparano, "Targeting Insulin Inhibition as a Metabolic Therapy in Advanced Cancer: A Pilot Safety and Feasibility Dietary Trial in 10 Patients", *Nutrition* 28(10) (2012), 1028–1035.

ACKNOWLEDGMENTS

Although my name is on the cover of this book, a project of this scope is always a team effort. I worked hand in glove with writer Olivia Bell Buehl, with whom I have collaborated many times. She takes my thoughts and words and polishes them until they gleam. Recipe developer Jennifer Iserloh, aka the Skinny Chef, created the quick and easy and Atkins-friendly recipes. Another Jennifer, Ms Knollenberg, developed the meal plans and did the nutritional analysis of the recipes to ensure their compliance with the New Atkins Diet.

Literary agent Joy Tutela of the David Black Agency was with us all the way from the moment we began to ask ourselves the question: How can we bring a new generation of people into the Atkins fold by making the diet easier than ever to understand and follow? Consultant and strategist Marc E. Jaffe, who knows everything there is to know about the book publishing business, brought his wealth of experience and sharp mind to the project.

Colleagues at Atkins Nutritionals also played crucial roles as we refined the editorial concept. Chief marketing executive Scott Parker reviewed multiple iterations of the manuscript and regularly challenged us to simplify, simplify, and further simplify both the diet and the language describing it. He also suggested using visual components wherever possible. Brand manager Nicole Thompson performed the Herculean task of keeping the various components moving forwards in sync, and on schedule, aided by assistant brand manager Carly

Hofstedt. Nutritionist Vicki Cuce acted as my right hand, cheerfully researching and resolving countless questions and issues.

My good friend and associate Jeff S. Volek, PhD, RD, one of the authors of *The New Atkins for a New You*, of which this book is an offshoot, wrote the chapter on the science attesting to the benefits of eating the low-carb way. Thank you, Jeff, for taking time away from your research on low-carb nutrition and fitness at the University of Connecticut.

Another shout-out goes to the nine Atkins followers who invited us into their lives and shared their amazing success stories. You are an inspiration to all of us who worked on this book and undoubtedly will equally inspire its readers.

Finally, thank you to our meticulous and insightful editor, Michelle Howry, and the rest of the editorial and production staff at Touchstone. With the publication of our fourth book, I can happily say that our working relationship is stronger than ever.

Colette Heimowitz

INDEX

Also available:

The New Atkins, New You Cookbook

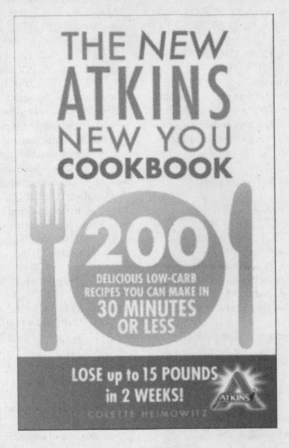

If you'd like more delicious Atkins-friendly recipes you'll love our cookbook. Includes satisfying and healthy low-carb ideas you can make in 30 minutes or less.

£10.99   ISBN: 9780091947521

For the latest information, tips and advice, visit The New Atkins website at http://uk.atkins.com/ and join our Atkins community on Facebook.